Modern Survival Analysis in Clinical Research

Ton J. Cleophas • Aeilko H. Zwinderman

Modern Survival Analysis in Clinical Research

Cox Regressions Versus Accelerated Failure Time Models

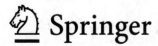 Springer

Ton J. Cleophas
Albert Schweitzer Hospital
Department Medicine
Dordrecht, Zuid-Holland
The Netherlands

Aeilko H. Zwinderman
Department Biostatistics and Epidemiology
Academic Medical Center
Amsterdam, Noord-Holland
The Netherlands

ISBN 978-3-031-31634-0   ISBN 978-3-031-31632-6   (eBook)
https://doi.org/10.1007/978-3-031-31632-6

This Springer imprint is published by the registered company Springer Nature Switzerland AG
The registered company address is: Gewerbestrasse 11, 6330 Cham, Switzerland

Preface

IBM (International Business Machines) has published in the 2023 version of its SPSS statistical software an important novel menu for Survival Analysis entitled Accelerated Failure Time (AFT) Models. Unlike the traditional Cox proportional hazard methods, the novel AFT Models predict the *times* of death rather than the *hazards* of death.

Although immensely popular, Cox regression has the problem that it is based on exponential models where per time unit the same percentage has an event, a pretty strong assumption for complex creatures like humans. Yet it has been widely used for the comparison of Kaplan Meier curves, simply because no better alternatives were obvious. In 1991, LJ Wei from Harvard Public Health School demonstrated that AFT models were a more useful alternative to Cox regression because it was less affected by omitting covariances and changing frequency distributions (Stat Med 1992: 11; 1871).

This was underscored in 1997 by N Keiding et al., statisticians from Copenhagen University, who also showed better-sensitive goodness of fit and null hypothesis tests with AFT than with Cox survival tests. In the past 20 years, AFT tests have started to being used not only in cancer research, public health studies, demographic and aging research, but also in reliability studies of industrial products, engineering studies, particularly those of steel and concrete superstructures, and many more fields. Studies were sometimes published in high impact journals like *Nature* (5x) and *Science* (7x).

So far, a controlled study of a representative sample of clinical Kaplan Meier assessments, where the sensitivity of Cox regression is systematically tested against that of AFT modeling, has not been accomplished. This edition is the first textbook and tutorial of AFT modeling for medical and healthcare students as well as recollection/update bench and help desk for professionals. Each chapter can be studied as a standalone, and, using, real as well as hypothesized data, it tests the performance of the novel methodology against traditional Cox regressions. Step-by-step analyses of over 20 data files stored at Supplementary Files at Springer Interlink are included for self-assessment.

We should add that the authors are well qualified in their field. Professor Zwinderman is past-president of the International Society of Biostatistics (2012–2015) and Professor Cleophas is past-president of the American College of Angiology (2000–2002). From their expertise, they should be able to make adequate selections of modern data analysis methods for the benefit of physicians, students, and investigators. The authors have been working and publishing together for 25 years, and their research can be characterized as a continued effort to demonstrate that clinical data analysis is not mathematics but rather a discipline at the interface of biology and mathematics.

Dordrecht, Zuid-Holland, The Netherlands

Ton J. Cleophas

Amsterdam, Noord-Holland, The Netherlands

Aeilko H. Zwinderman

Contents

Chapter 1
Regression Analysis

Abstract Students in medicine and health sciences find regression analyses harder than any other methodology in statistics. This edition will start with a brief review of history, and methodologies of regression analyses. Linear regression has a continuous outcome variable. In contrast, logistic and Cox regressions have binary outcomes, and use logarithmic transformations of odds or hazards. This edition will particularly focus on the novel models for survival analysis entitled Accelerated failure times models, that provide generally better data-fit than does the traditional Cox regressions based on odds of events, here otherwise called hazard of events, particularly if the events are nasty.

1.1 Introduction

The authors as professors in statistics and machine learning at European universities are worried, that their students find regression analyses harder than any other methodology in statistics. This edition will start with a brief review of history, and methodologies. Then we will focus on the novel models for survival analysis entitled Accelerated failure times models.

1.2 History

The earliest form of regression, called the least squares method, was invented around 1800, by Legendre (1752–1833), a mathematician from Paris, and Gauss (1777–1855), a mathematician from Göttingen Germany. Quetelet from Belgium (1796–1874) worked and later published with Legendre. Initially, only continuous outcome variables were assessed. However, already in the 1830s and 40s regression models with binary rather than continuous outcome variables were subject of statistical research. The logistic function was developed as a model of population growth and named "logistic" by Pierre François Verhulst (1804–1849), a Belgian student,

T. J. Cleophas, A. H. Zwinderman, *Modern Survival Analysis in Clinical Research*, https://doi.org/10.1007/978-3-031-31632-6_1

and, later, a close colleague of Quetelet. He was well aware, that the logistic model was based on exponential relationships, and lead often to impossible values, and that some kind of adjustment was required. Like Quetelet, he approached the problem of population growth by adding extra terms to the logistic model-equation. Another important regression model with binary outcome is Cox regression developed many years later than logistic regression by David Cox from Birmingham UK (1928–2016). He viewed survival models as consistent of two parts: first the underlying baseline hazard function describing, how the risk of event per time unit changed over time, and, second, the effect parameters, describing, how the hazard varied in response to explanatory covariates. A typical medical example would include covariates, like treatment assignment, as well as patient characteristics, like patient age at the start of a study, gender, and the presence of other diseases at the start of a study, in order to reduce variability and/or control for confounding. He viewed survival models as consistent of two parts: first the underlying baseline hazard function describing, how the risk of event per time unit changed over time, and, second, the effect parameters, describing, how the hazard varied in response to explanatory covariates. A typical medical example would include covariates like treatment assignment, as well as patient characteristics like patient age at the start of a study, gender, and the presence of other diseases, in order to reduce variability and control for confounding.

1.3   Methodologies of Regression Analysis

1.3.1   Linear Regression

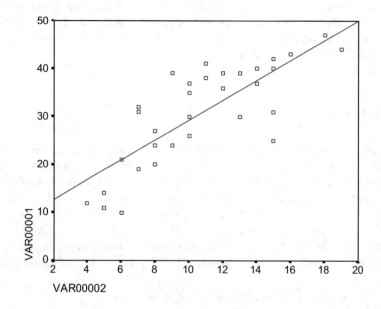

The above graph shows the data of a crossover study of the effect of an old laxative (bisacodyl) on a novel one. Bisacodyl is plotted along the x-axis, the new laxative along the y-axis.

The graph shows that something special is going on: the data are closer to the line than could happen by chance. The diagonal line is the best fit line of the data, i.e., there is no better line, no closer to the data. The line shows a positive correlation between the two variables and is drawn according to the equation $y = a + bx$. For every x-value the line provides the best predictable y-value in the population. y is the dependent variable, x the independent variable, b the regression coefficient (= direction coefficient), and a the intercept (the place where the line crosses the y-axis). The a and b values can be computed by heart, but this is a lot of work and much easier is to use a software program for the purpose.

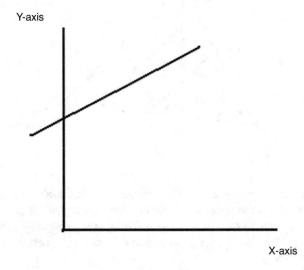

A simple linear regression uses the equation $y = a + bx$. The equation is applied for making predictions from the -values about the y-values.

If we fill out the   x-value   = 0, the equation will turn into $y = a$,
                   x   = 1 $y = a + b$
                   x   = 2 $y = a + 2b$.

For each x-value the equation gives the best predictable y-value, all of the y-values constitute a line = best fit line for the data (with the shortest distance of x-values from y-values).

With multiple variables regression with three variables the equation used is $y = a + b_1 x_1 + b_2 x_2$.

A 3 axes model with y-axis, x_1-axis and x_2-axis can be used for imaging:

If we fill out $x_1 = 0$, the equation will turn into $y = a + b_2 x_2$
                     $x_1 = 1$, the equation will turn into $y = a + b_1 + b_2 x_2$
                     $x_1 = 2$, the equation will turn into $y = a + 2b_1 + b_2 x_2$
                     $x_1 = 3$, the equation will turn into $y = a + 3b_1 + b_2 x_2$.

Each x_1-value has its own regression line and all of the lines constitute regression planes, which are the best fit plane of the data in space (with the shortest distance of the x-values from the y-values).

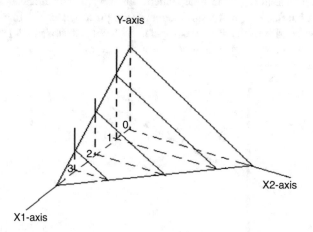

With more than 3 variables the data model is multidimensional and beyond imagination, but for a computer this is no problem. Computations about distances and uncertainties can be readily performed. Multiple variables regression are fine for determining statistically significant predictor variables, otherwise called independent predictors.

Linear regressions use continuous x and y variables. However, instead of a continuous x variable, also a binary x variable is possible. An example is given underneath. A parallel group study of 872 patients compared the efficacy on LDL cholesterol levels of placebo and pravastatin. An unpaired T-test was used for statistical testing.

N = sample size, SD = standard deviation, SEM = standard error of the mean.

	Placebo	pravastatin	difference
n	434	438	
mean	−0.04	1.23	1.27
SD	0.59	0.68	SEM = 0.043

The same results can be obtained by drawing the best fit data in the form of a regression line. The underneath graph gives the results from a regression analysis. The x variable has only 2 values, 0 or 1, 0 means placebo, 1 means pravastatin.

The regression coefficient b is equal to 1,27, which is identical to the difference of two means. The regression coefficient b has an SE (standard error) identical to that of the pooled sum of the SEs of the two means. Particularly in clinical research x variables are often binary and regressions are a very convenient method for analysis even with multiple x variables. Binary predictor variables will be applied in many chapters of the current edition.

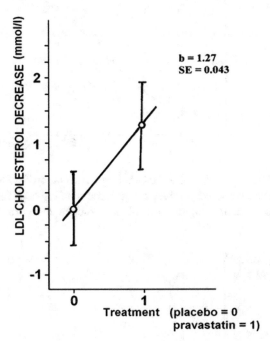

1.3.2 Logistic Regression

With logistic regression the dependent variable is not continuous, like the above y-values but rather binary, meaning that they can only adopt two outcomes: yes or no.

For example, the odds of an infarction could be the outcome. The outcome values are then yes or no. The odds of infarction in a population is the ratio of

$$\frac{\text{number of patients with}}{\text{number of patients without}}.$$

Clinically we suspect, that the odds of infarction is correlated with age. But we do not know how.

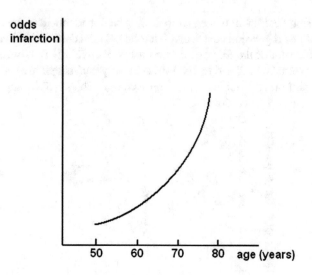

Experimentally, it can be observed that the correlation is not linear at all. However, when the measured y-values are replaced with log odds (or rather ln odds values where ln = natural logarithm), all of a sudden the correlation seems to be linear.

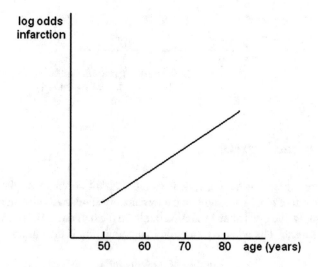

And so, when we transform

$$y = a + bx$$

into a loglinear model

$$\text{ln odds} = a + bx \text{ where } x = \text{age variable,}$$

then a handsome model for making predictions about the risk of infarction from the years of age is obtained.

In SPSS statistical software:

Command:
click binary logistic regression.....click dependent variable: for infarct yes or no enter 1 or 0.....click independent variable: enter years of age.

In the output the best fit a and b values from the equation $y = a + bx$ will be given.

$$a = -9.2$$

$$b = 0.1 (\text{SE} = 0.04; \text{p} < 0.05),$$

which means that data are closer to the regression curve than could happen by chance. Age is, therefore, a significant determinant of the odds of infarct ($\approx$ risk of infarct).

We can use the equation to predict odds of infarction from a patient's age:

$$\text{Ln odds at 55 years} = -9.2 + 0.1 \quad .55 = -4.82265$$
$$\text{odds} \qquad\qquad = 0.008$$
$$\qquad\qquad = 8 / 1000$$

$$\text{Ln odds at 75 years} = -9.2 + 0.1 \quad .75 = -1.3635$$
$$\text{odds} \qquad\qquad = 0.256$$
$$\qquad\qquad = 256 / 1000$$

At the age of seventy-five the risk of infarction will be over 30 times larger than it will at the age of fifty-five.

The odds of infarction can be more accurately be predicted, when multiple x-variables are used. Also, logistic regression can be used to test whether two different predictors like treatment modalities or age classes are significantly different from one another.

1.3.3   Cox Regression

Cox regressions are immensely popular for survival analysis. With survival or death data, just like with logistic regression, no linear relationship exists between the predictor, the time, and the outcome. The proportion of survivors or that of deaths.

The outcome proportion of deaths is estimated with odds, with deaths otherwise called hazard. Unfortunately, this hazard model tends to provide poor data-fits. The novel Accelerated failure time models work with chances and provide a better data-fit than does the odds methodology. In the Chaps. 2 and 3 explanations will be given, in the Chaps. 4, 5, 6, 7, 8, 9, 10, 11, 12, 13, 14, 15, 16, 17, 18, 19, 20 and 21 of this edition many examples will further explain the differences between Cox regression and Accelerated failure time analysis methods.

1.4   Conclusion

Students in medicine and health sciences find regression analyses harder than any other methodology in statistics. This edition gives a brief review of history, and methodologies. Linear regression has a continuous outcome variable. In contrast, logistic and Cox regressions have a binary outcome, and uses logarithmic transformations of odds or hazards of events. This edition will particularly focus on the novel models for survival analysis entitled Accelerated failure times models, that provide generally better data-fit than does the traditional Cox regressions based on odds of events here often otherwise called hazard of events, particularly if the event is something nasty.

References

Five textbooks complementary to the current production and written by the same authors are
(1) Statistics applied to clinical studies 5th edition, 2012,
(2) Machine learning in medicine a complete overview, 2020,
(3) Regression Analysis in Medical Research, 2nd Edition, 2021,
(4) Quantile Regression in Clinical Research, 2021,
(5) Kernel Ridge Regression in Clinical Research, 2022,
all of them edited by Springer Heidelberg Germany.

Chapter 2
Cox Regressions

Abstract The Chaps. 1, 2, and 3 of this edition will review the general principles of the most popular regression models in a nonmathematical fashion, including linear regression, the main purposes of regression analyses, the methods of logistic regression for event analysis, and Cox regression for hazard analysis. Cox regression is just like logistic regression immensely popular in clinical research. It is based on exponential-like models: per time unit the same % of patients has an event.

2.1 Introduction

Regression analysis is harder to make students understand than any other methodology in statistics. Particularly, medical and health care students rapidly get lost, because of dependent data and covariances, that must be accounted all the time. The problem is, that high school algebra is familiar with equations like $y = a + b\,x$, but it never addresses equations like $y = a + b_1\,x_1 + b_2\,x_2$, let alone $y = a + b_1\,x_1 + b_2\,x_2 + b_1\,x_1 \cdot b_2\,x_2$. In the past 30 years the theoretical basis of regression analysis has changed little, but the EMA has just decided to include directives regarding the baseline characteristics in the statistical analysis of controlled clinical trials. Regression methods have, thus, obtained a reason for existence in this field, while a short time ago their use was limited to hypothesis-generating rather than hypothesis-testing research. The Chaps. 1, 2, and 3 will review the general principles of the most popular regression models in a nonmathematical fashion, including linear regression, the main purposes of regression analyses, the methods of logistic regression for event analysis, and Cox regression for hazard analysis. Cox regression is just like logistic regression immensely popular in clinical research. It is based on an exponential model: per time unit the same % of patients has an event.

T. J. Cleophas, A. H. Zwinderman, *Modern Survival Analysis in Clinical Research*, https://doi.org/10.1007/978-3-031-31632-6_2

2.2   History of Cox Regressions

An important regression model with binary outcome is Cox regression developed many years later than logistic regression by David Cox from Birmingham UK (1928–2016). He viewed survival models as consistent of two parts: first the underlying baseline hazard function describing, how the risk of event per time unit changed over time, and, second, the effect parameters, describing, how the hazard varied in response to explanatory covariates. A typical medical example would include covariates, like treatment assignment, as well as patient characteristics, like patient age at the start of a study, gender, and the presence of other diseases at the start of a study, in order to reduce variability and/or control for confounding. He viewed survival models as consistent of two parts: first the underlying baseline hazard function describing, how the risk of event per time unit changed over time, and, second, the effect parameters, describing, how the hazard varied in response to explanatory covariates. A typical medical example would include covariates, like treatment assignment, as well as patient characteristics, like patient age at the start of a study, gender, and the presence of other diseases at the start of a study, in order to reduce variability and/or control for confounding.

2.3   Principles of Cox Regressions

Another regression model is just like logistic regression immensely popular in clinical research. That is Cox regression. It is based on an exponential model: per time unit the same % of patients has an event, which is a pretty strong assumption for complex creatures like man. Exponential models may be adequate for mosquitos, but less so for human creatures. Yet Cox regressions are widely used for comparisons of Kaplan-Meier curves in humans.

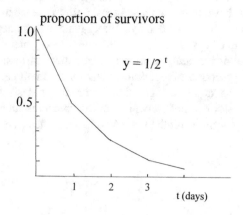

Cox uses an exponential model. Above an example is given of mosquitos in a room with concrete walls. They only die when colliding against the concrete wall. Unlike with complex creatures like humans there are no other reasons for dying. In this setting a survival half life can be pretty easily computed. In the above example, after one day 50% of the mosquitos are alive, after the second day 25% etc. A mathematical equation for proportion survivors $= (1/2)^t = 2^{-t}$. In true biology the e value 2.71828 better fits the data than does 2, and k is applied as a constant for the species. In this way the proportion survivors can be expressed as

$$\text{proportion survivors} = e^{-kt}$$

Underneath an example is given of Kaplan-Meier curves in humans, and their exponential best fit Cox models, the dotted lines.

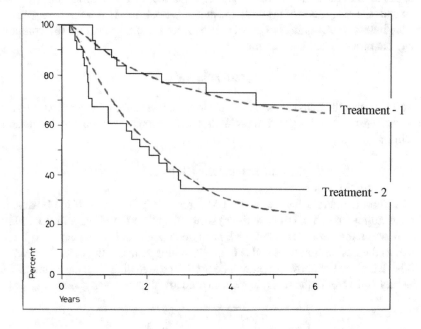

The equations of the Cox models run like:

$$\text{proportion survivors} = e^{-kt-bx}$$

x = a binary variable (only 0 or 1, 0 means treatment 1, 1 means treatment 2), b = the regression coefficient. If x = 0, then the equation turns into.

$$\text{proportion survivors} = e^{-kt}$$

If x = 1, then the equation turns into.

$$\text{proportion survivors} = e^{-kt-b}$$

Now, the relative chance of survival is given.

$$\text{relative chance of survival} = e^{-kt-b} / e^{-kt}$$
$$= e^{-b}$$

and, likewise, the relative chance of death = 1/e to the power b.

We should add here that in the past computers did not easily run on proportions of survivors that have a very small interval between 0 and 1 (= unit = 100%). And in practice they have been replaced with odds of survivors = number of survivors/ number of non-survivors. With death as outcome the term odds has been replaced with the term hazard but the meaning is equal to that of odds. Unfortunately with large odds the magnitude of the odds and that of the risk gets increasingly unprecise, but nontheless when talking of hazard or proportional hazard ratios we still continue to call the proportional hazard ratio.

$$\text{hazard ratio} = e^{b}.$$

Just like with the odds ratios used in the logistic regressions, the hazard ratios are analyzed with natural logarithmic (ln) transformations, because the ln hazards are linear.

$$\text{ln hazard ratio}(HR) = b$$

The computer can calculate the best fit b for a data file given. If the b value is significantly >0, then the HR (= antiln b) is significantly >1, and a significant difference between the hazard of death is between treatment 2 and 1. The hazard is interpreted as the risk similar to the odds of an event interpreted as the risk of an event.

The data from the above graph will be used for a statistical analysis using SPSS statistical software. In the results sheets the underneath table was given:

b	standard error	t	p
1.10	0.41	2.68	0.01

The hazard ratio of treatment 2 versus treatment 1 ad given equals $e^{b} = e^{1.10} = 3.00$. This hazard ratio is significantly larger than 1 at p = 0.01. Thus, the treatments are significantly different from one another. For statistical testing the significance of difference between the risks of death between two treatments also a chi-square test can be applied. It would produce an even better p-value of 0.002. However, Cox regression can adjust for subgroups, like relevant prognostic factors, and chi-square tests cannot do so. For example, the hazard of death in the above example could be influenced by the disease stage, and by the presence of B-symptoms. If these data are in the data file, then the analysis can be extended according to the underneath model.

$$HR = e^{b1\,x1 + b2\,x2 + b3\,x3}$$

All of the x-variables are binary.

$x_1 = 0$ means treatment 1, $x_1 = 1$ means treatment 2.
$x_2 = 0$ means disease stage I–III, $x_2 = 1$ means disease stage IV.
$x_3 = 0$ means A symptoms, $x_3 = 1$ means B symptoms.

The data file is entered in the SPSS software program, and commands similar to the above ones are given.

The underneath table is in the output sheets.

Covariate	b	standard error	p-value
treatment modality(x_1)	1.10	0.45	< 0.05
disease stage(x_2)	1.38	0.55	< 0.05
symptoms(x_3)	1.74	0.69	< 0.05

HR of treatment 2 versus 1	$= e^{1.10} = 3.00$
HR of disease stage IV versus I-III	$= e^{1.38} = 3.97$
HR of B-symptoms versus A-symptoms	$= e^{1.74} = 5.70$
The HR adjusted for treatment, disease stage and B-symptoms	$= e^{1.10 + 1.38 + 1.74} = 68.00$.

We can conclude that the treatment-2, after adjustment for disease stage IV and b-symptoms, raises a 68 higher mortality than does the treatment-1 without adjustments.

We need to account some of the problems with Cox regressions. Cox regression is a major simplification of biological processes. It is less sensitive than the chi-square test, it massages data (the above modeled Kaplan-Meier curves showed that few died within first 8 months, and that they continued to die after 2½ years??!!). Also a HR of 68 seems clinically unrealistically large. Clinicians know darn well that the disease stage and the presence of B symptoms must interact with one another on the outcome. In addition, Cox regression produces exponential types of relationships only.

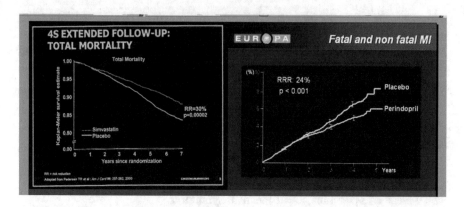

The above graphs from famous international mortality studies show that Cox regression analysis has sometimes been inadequately applied. It is inadequate, if a treatment effect only starts after 1–2 years, or if it starts immediately like with coronary interventions, or if unexpected effects start to interfere like with graph versus host effects.

One final point is that of censored data. The survival analysis has two types of patients stopping participation. One is death or any other event, the other is stopping participation for any reason but not because of an event. A censored patient is a patient whose days in the study is accounted but no event is counted in the outcome. In many chapter of this edition censored patients will be observed.

2.4   Conclusion

Regression analysis is harder to make students understand than any other methodology in statistics. Particularly, medical and health care students rapidly get lost, because of dependent data and covariances, that must be accounted all the time. The problem is, that high school algebra is familiar with equations like $y = a + b\,x$, but it never addresses equations like $y = a + b_1\,x_1 + b_2\,x_2$, let alone $y = a + b_1\,x_1 + b_2\,x_2 + b_1\,x_1 \cdot b_2\,x_2$. In the past 30 years the theoretical basis of regression analysis has changed little, but the EMA has just decided to include directives regarding the baseline characteristics in the statistical analysis of controlled clinical trials. Regression methods have, thus, obtained a reason for existence in this field, while a short time ago their use was limited to hypothesis-generating rather than hypothesis-testing research.

The Chaps. 1, 2, and 3 review the general principles of the most popular regression models in a nonmathematical fashion, including simple and multiple linear regression, the main purposes of regression analyses, the methods of logistic regression for event analysis, and Cox regression for hazard analysis. Just like with previous editions of the authors, e.g., "Understanding clinical data analysis, learning statistical principles from published clinical research, Springer Heidelberg Germany,

2017", particular attention has been given to common sense rationing and more intuitive explanations of the pretty complex statistical methodologies, rather than bloodless algebraic proofs of the methods.

Finally, the explorative nature of regression analysis must be emphasized. In our edition 2012 edition Statistics applied to clinical studies 5th edition we stated as follows. There is always an air of uncertainty with regression analysis. Regression in the context of clinical trials is exploratory mostly. Regression massages the data, and, thus, massages reality. It is incredible, that regression, nonetheless, took so much possession of clinical trials. Generally, you should interpret regression analysis as interesting, but an analysis that proves nothing. Today, 10 years later, regression is getting more mature, and is increasingly accepted for the analysis of controlled clinical trials. However, limitations must be mentioned. In controlled clinical trials only a single covariate like a baseline characteristic is recommended by drug administrations like the European Medicines Administration.

References

Five textbooks complementary to the current production and written by the same authors are
(1) Statistics applied to clinical studies 5th edition, 2012,
(2) Machine learning in medicine a complete overview, 2020,
(3) Regression Analysis in Medical Research, 2nd Edition, 2021,
(4) Quantile Regression in Clinical Research, 2021,
(5) Kernel Ridge Regression in Clinical Research, 2022,
all of them edited by Springer Heidelberg Germany.

Chapter 3
Accelerated Failure Time Models

Abstract Accelerated failure time models do not use, like Cox regression (Chap. 1), the hazard of death, but, rather, the risk of death. The hazard is the ratio "death/non-deaths", while the risk of death is the ratio "death/entire population at the start of a study". The hazard runs from zero to $+\infty$, whereas the risk runs from zero to 1 (= 100%). Both hazard and risk modeling can be accomplished with mathematical functions that are even largely similar. For the purpose of optimized fitting the relationships between time and survival risk and their relative risks five options may be chosen:

1. Weibull models
2. Exponential models
3. Log-normal models
4. Log-logistic models
5. Hypertabastic models based on hyperbolic secants, i.e., the inverse of hyperbolic cosines.

Mathematical models are for finding and fitting significant relationships between predictor and outcome variables and traditional tests are usually applied for testing how far distant the data are from the best fit models. The closer they are, the better suited the models are for predictive purposes, like times to event, survival, death, failures.

3.1 Introduction

Accelerated failure time models do not use, like Cox regression (Chap. 1), the hazard of death, but, rather, the risk of death. The hazard is the ratio "death/non-deaths", while the risk of death is the ratio "death/entire population at the start of a study". The hazard runs from zero to $+\infty$, whereas the risk runs from zero to 1 (= 100%). Both hazard and risk modeling can be accomplished with mathematical functions that are even largely similar. IBM (international Business machines) has published in its SPSS statistical software 2023 update (version 29) a new addition to its menu

T. J. Cleophas, A. H. Zwinderman, *Modern Survival Analysis in Clinical Research*, https://doi.org/10.1007/978-3-031-31632-6_3

module Survival Analysis entitled Accelerated Failure Time (AFT) Models. Whereas the traditional method for survival analysis, i.e., Cox Proportional Hazard Analysis, assumes, that a predictor variable affects the hazard of death, the AFT (accelerated failure time) models, in contrast, only assumes, that a predictor variable affects the time of death. Although immensely popular, many problems with it have been widely recognized and it has, therefore, even been named a "major simplification of nature", where per time unit the same percentage of subjects will die. This may be closely true for simple creatures like mosquitos but less so for complex creatures like human beings suffering from confoundings and interactions all the time. AFT models try and fit survival data using, instead of the log odds of surviving (= hazard of surviving), the proportion of survivors (= risk of surviving). While the former runs from minus ∞ to plus ∞, the latter runs from minus 1 to plus 1. With the latter analyses statistical software tended to get stuck due to narrow computational intervals in the past. But, with current logarithmic transformations monotonous increasing or decreasing mathematical functions have been successfully used. Particularly, prior knowledge about the patterns to be expected is helpful here. And if this is not available, "trial and error" methods can be recommended, i.e., logarithmic transformations of either the x- or the y-axis or both of them. For the purpose of optimized fitting the relationships between time and survival risk and their relative risks five options are may be chosen:

1. Weibull models
2. Exponential models
3. Log-normal models
4. Log-logistic models
5. Hypertabastic models based on hyperbolic secants, i.e., the inverse of hyperbolic cosines.

Mathematical models are for finding and fitting significant relationships between predictor and outcome variables and traditional tests are usually applied for testing how far distant the data are from the best fit models. The closer they are, the better suited the models are for predictive purposes, like times to event, survival, death, failures.

3.2   History of Failure Time Models

IBM (International Business Machines) has published in the 2023 version of its SPSS statistical software an important novel menu for Survival Analysis entitled Accelerated Failure Time (AFT) models. Unlike the traditional Cox proportional hazard methods, the novel AFT Models predict the *times* of death rather than the *hazards* of death.

Although immensely popular, Cox regression has the problem that it is based on exponential models where per time unit the same percentage has an event, a pretty strong assumption for complex creatures like humans. Yet it has been widely used for the comparison of Kaplan Meier curves, simply because no better alternatives were obvious. In 1991 LJ Wei from Harvard Public Health School demonstrated, that AFT models were a more useful alternative to Cox regression, because it was less affected by omitting covariances and changing frequency distributions (Stat Med 1992: 11; 1871).

This was underscored in 1997 by N Keiding et al., statisticians from Copenhagen University, who also showed better-sensitive goodness of fit and null hypothesis tests with AFT than with Cox survival tests. In the past 20 years AFT tests have started to being used not only in cancer research, public health studies, demographic and aging research, but also in reliability studies of industrial products, engineering studies, particularly those of steel and concrete superstructures, and many more fields. Studies were sometimes published in high impact journals like Nature (5x) and Science (7x).

So far, a controlled study of a representative sample of clinical Kaplan Meier assessments, where the sensitivity of Cox regression is systematically tested against that of AFT modeling, has not been accomplished. This edition is the first textbook and tutorial of AFT modeling for medical and healthcare students as well as recol-lection/update bench, and help desk for professionals. Each chapter can be studied as a standalone, and, using, real as well as hypothesized data, it tests the perfor-mance of the novel methodology against traditional Cox regressions. Step by step analyses of 20 data files stored at Supplementary Files at Springer Interlink are included for self-assessment.

3.3   Methodology of Failure Time Models

Accelerated failure time models do not use, like Cox regression (Chap. 1), the haz-ard of death, but, rather, the risk of death. The hazard is the ratio "death/non-deaths", while the risk of death is the ratio "death/entire population at the start of a study". The hazard runs from zero to $+ \infty$, whereas the risk runs from zero to 1 ($= 100\%$). Both hazard and risk modeling can be assessed with exponential mathematical functions that are even similar.

For example, a simple function for hazard models is given by
hazard of surviving $= e^{-kt - bx}$ (see Chap. 1)
hazard ratio $= e^{b}$ (see Chap. 1)

For example, a simple function for chance models otherwise called risk models is given by
chance of surviving $= e^{-kt - bx}$
chance ratio (or risk) ratio $= e^{b}$

However, as hazards cover much larger intervals than risks do, fitting the latter to mathematical functions is harder, and special logarithmic transformations are

required for the models to better fit experimental data. Successful logarithmic transformations for accelerated failure time models are:

1. Weibull distribution
2. Exponential distribution
3. Log normal distribution
4. Log logistic distribution
5. Hypertabastic distribution (including hyperbolics in its function).

How does fitting work?

The general principle of regression analysis is applied: regression-analysis calculates best fit "line/exp-curve/curvilinear-curve" (the one with the shortest distance from data) and tests how far distant from curve the data are. A significant
correlation between y- and x-data means that the y data are closer to best fit data
model than will happen with random sampling. Statistical testing is usually performed with simple tests like the t-test, or analysis of variance. The "model-
principle" is fascinating but at the same time the largest limitation of regression
analysis, because it is often no use forcing nature into a mathematical model.

With survival analysis, either Cox or Accelerated failure time models, Kaplan
Meier graphs are first drawn of the data. Then regression curves are estimated making use of iterations (guesstimated), and the one with the best fit is chosen.

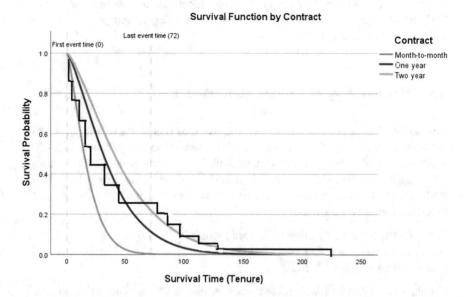

The above curves show an example taken from "What's new in IBM Statistics
version 29 published in 2023". We drew the graph in black as a hypothesized example of a Kaplan-Meier curve. With the help of mathematical functions (in color) the
best fit predictive model can be identified. Ordinary least square computations are
adequate for testing the distances of the data from the predictive model.

Why is the novel methodology called *accelerated* failure time modeling? In the above figure three best fit curves are given, and a Kaplan-Meier curve is drawn in black. Of the three best fit curves the left end curve provides a survival time of only ≈ 70 days versus ≈130 and ≈170 days of the other two curves. The left end curve provides not only a best fit curve but also, and at the same time, it provides the shortest survival time. This is the reason for the name of the methodology.

What does the Akaike information criterion say? Most mathematical models in biomedicine have considerable residual scatter around the regression line, and the Akaike information criterion (AIC) is a measure of the relative goodness of fit of a mathematical model for describing the trade off between bias and variance in model construction, and to assess the accuracy of the regression model used. However, the AIC, as it is a relative measure, will not be helpful to confirm a good result, if all of the regression models fit the dataset poorly.

Mathematical functions may, thus, provide an adequate fit for one or more Kaplan Meier survival curves. And with accelerated failure time models the so called Weibull equation with k and λ as shape and scale parameters is a good example of such a function.

The Weibull Probability density function

$$f(x) = \frac{k}{\lambda}\left(\frac{x}{\lambda}\right)^{k-1} e^{-(x/\lambda)^k}$$

With k = 1, λ = 1 and x > 0 the above equation reduces to f (x) = e^{-x}.
The underneath graph shows the mathematical curve of the above function.

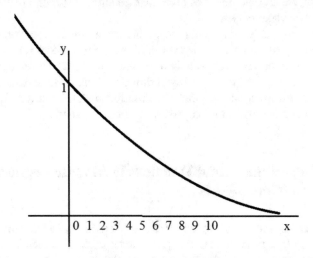

With f (x) = y = survival probability (S) and x = t = time to event, the curve looks like a Weibull survival function.

$$S(t) = e^{-t}$$

For assessment effect of, for example, a treatment modality on the outcome survival probability a novel x – variable must be added to the equation.
The underneath equation shows that bx is added for the purpose.

$$S(t) = e^{-t+bx}$$

x = variable treatment modality. It has only two values: a zero for treatment II, and a one for treatment I.

With treatment I the equation changes into $S(t) = e^{-t+b}$
With treatment II $S(t) = e^{-t}$

The function for relative chance of death (or relative risk ratio) changes accordingly

$$\text{Relative risk ratio} = \frac{e^{-t+b}}{e^{-t}} = e^{b}$$

ln (natural logarithm) of $e^{b} = b$
ln of risk ratio is thus b, otherwise called the regression coefficient of the regression equation.

Instead of Weibull distributions other mathematical distributions may better fit various Kaplan-Meier curves.

Cox may adequately work using the simple hazard model function which runs with a wide interval from 0 to ∞. However, fitting the risk model is harder, because it runs with a very narrow interval only from 0 to 1 (= 100%). Different mathematical functions are required for a successful fitting of Kaplan-Meier data. Particularly logarithmic transformations are often required for models to fit data successfully. Underneath the graphs of some successful functions are shown.

3.4   Graphs of Successful Functions to Analyze Accelerated Failure Time Models

Graphs of some successful functions as applied in the SPSS menu entitled Accelerated failure time models are given underneath. For each function curve some intervals are applicable for fitting Kaplan-Meier curves.

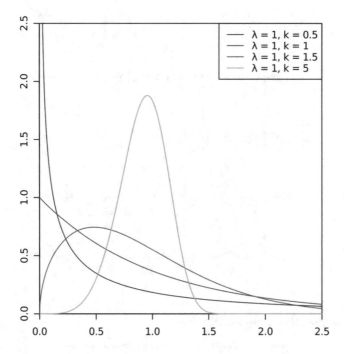

Weibull Frequency Distribution with on the x-axis f.e. time (t) and on the y-axis f.e. probability or chance or hazard of survival S(t).

$$S(t) = e^{-\lambda(t^k)}$$

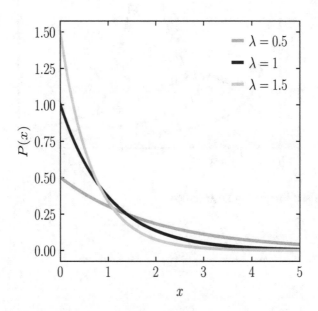

Exponential Frequency Distribution

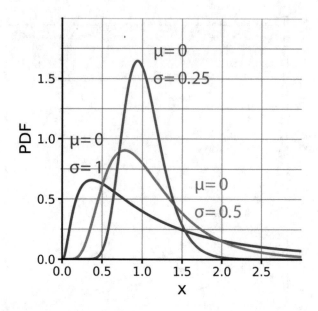

Log Normal Frequency Distribution

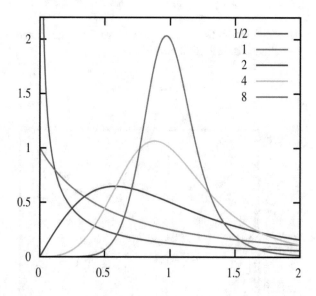

Log Logistic Frequency Distribution

3.5 Conclusion

Accelerated failure time models do not use, like Cox regression (Chap. 1), the hazard of death, but, rather, the risk of death. The hazard is the ratio "death/non-deaths", while the risk of death is the ratio "death/entire population at the start of a study". The hazard runs from zero to ∞, whereas the risk runs from zero to 1 (= 100%). Both hazard and risk modeling can be accomplished with mathematical functions that are even largely similar. For example, a simple function for hazard models is given by

hazard of surviving = $e^{-kt\,-bx}$ (see Chap. 1)
hazard ratio = e^b (see Chap.1)

For example, a simple function for chance otherwise called risk models is given by

chance of surviving = $e^{-kt\,-bx}$
and chance ratio (or risk) ratio = e^b.

However, as hazards cover much larger intervals than risks do, fitting the latter to mathematical functions is harder, and special logarithmic transformations are required for the models to fit experimental data successfully. Successful logarithmic transformations for accelerated failure time models are:

1. Weibull distribution
2. Exponential distribution
3. Log normal distribution
4. Log logistic distribution
5. Hypertabastic distribution (including hyperbolics in its function).

How does fitting work?

The general principle of regression analysis is applied: regression-analysis calculates best fit "line/exponential-curve/curvilinear-curve" (the ones with the shortest distance from data) and tests how far distant from curves the data are. A significant correlation between y and x-data means that the y data are closer to model than will happen with random sampling. Statistical testing is usually performed with simple tests like the t-test, or analysis of variance. The "model-principle" is fascinating but at the same time the largest limitation of regression analysis, because it is often no use forcing nature into a model. With survival analysis using either Cox or Accelerated failure time models, Kaplan-Meier graphs are first drawn of the data. Then regression curves are estimated making use of iterations (guesstimated), and the one with the best fit is chosen.

References

Five textbooks complementary to the current production and written by the same authors are
(1) Statistics applied to clinical studies 5th edition, 2012,
(2) Machine learning in medicine a complete overview, 2020,
(3) Regression Analysis in Medical Research, 2nd Edition, 2021,
(4) Quantile Regression in Clinical Research, 2021,
(5) Kernel Ridge Regression in Clinical Research, 2022,
all of them edited by Springer Heidelberg Germany.

Chapter 4
Simple Dataset with Event as Outcome and Treatment as Predictor

Abstract In 60 patients with cardiovascular disease the treatment modality was a statistically significant predictor of event at a p-value of 0,004 in the Cox regression. With the Accelerated failure time model the p-value even fell to p = 0,001.

4.1 Introduction

There are often clinical arguments to support that medical treatments may influence survival. However documented proof is often missing. In this chapter the effect on survival of a novel treatment is assessed against a control treatment. Survival can be measured in the form of either a hazard, which is the ratio of deaths and non-deaths in a random sample, or as a risk which is the proportion of deaths in the same sample. In this chapter hazard and risk of the same data will be computed in a 60 patient parallel group study using respectively Cox regression and Accelerated failure time models.

4.2 Data Example

The underneath data are a summary of the study applied in this data example. Treat = treatment.

Supplementary Information The online version contains supplementary material available at https://doi.org/10.1007/978-3-031-31632-6_4.

T. J. Cleophas, A. H. Zwinderman, *Modern Survival Analysis in Clinical Research*, https://doi.org/10.1007/978-3-031-31632-6_4

27

time to event months	event 1 = yes	treat 0 or 1	age year	gender 0 = fem	LDL cholesterol
1,00	1	0	65,00	,00	2,00
1,00	1	0	66,00	,00	2,00
2,00	1	0	73,00	,00	2,00
2,00	1	0	54,00	,00	2,00
2,00	1	0	46,00	,00	2,00
2,00	1	0	37,00	,00	2,00
2,00	1	0	54,00	,00	2,00
2,00	1	0	66,00	,00	2,00
2,00	1	0	44,00	,00	2,00
3,00	0	0	62,00	,00	2,00
4,00	1	0	57,00	,00	2,00
5,00	1	0	43,00	,00	2,00
6,00	1	0	85,00	,00	2,00
6,00	1	0	46,00	,00	2,00
7,00	1	0	76,00	,00	2,00
9,00	1	0	76,00	,00	2,00
9,00	1	0	65,00	,00	1,00
11,00	1	0	54,00	,00	1,00
12,00	1	0	34,00	,00	1,00
14,00	1	0	45,00	,00	1,00
16,00	1	0	56,00	1,00	1,00
17,00	1	0	67,00	1,00	1,00
18,00	1	0	86,00	1,00	2,00
30,00	0	0	75,00	1,00	2,00
30,00	0	0	65,00	1,00	2,00
30,00	0	0	54,00	1,00	2,00
30,00	0	0	46,00	1,00	2,00
30,00	0	0	54,00	1,00	2,00
30,00	0	0	75,00	1,00	2,00
30,00	0	0	56,00	1,00	2,00
30,00	0	1	56,00	1,00	2,00
30,00	0	1	53,00	1,00	2,00
30,00	0	1	34,00	1,00	2,00
30,00	0	1	35,00	1,00	2,00
30,00	0	1	37,00	1,00	2,00
30,00	0	1	65,00	1,00	2,00
30,00	0	1	45,00	1,00	2,00
30,00	0	1	66,00	1,00	2,00
30,00	0	1	55,00	1,00	2,00
30,00	0	1	88,00	1,00	1,00
29,00	1	1	67,00	1,00	1,00
29,00	1	1	56,00	1,00	1,00
29,00	1	1	54,00	1,00	1,00

(continued)

time to event	event 1 =	treat 0	age	gender 0	LDL
months	yes	or 1	year	= fem	cholesterol
28,00	0	1	57,00	1,00	1,00
28,00	1	1	57,00	1,00	1,00
28,00	1	1	76,00	1,00	1,00
27,00	1	1	67,00	1,00	1,00
26,00	1	1	66,00	1,00	1,00
24,00	1	1	56,00	1,00	1,00
23,00	1	1	66,00	1,00	1,00
22,00	1	1	84,00	1,00	1,00
22,00	0	1	56,00	1,00	1,00
21,00	1	1	46,00	1,00	1,00
20,00	1	1	45,00	1,00	1,00
19,00	1	1	76,00	1,00	1,00
19,00	1	1	65,00	1,00	1,00
18,00	1	1	45,00	1,00	1,00
17,00	1	1	76,00	1,00	1,00
16,00	1	1	56,00	1,00	1,00
16,00	1	1	45,00	1,00	1,00

4.3   Data Analysis in SPSS Statistical Software Version 29

The commands for Cox regression and for Accelerated failure time models are summarized underneath.

For convenience the data file entitled "Chapter 4,......" is in SpringerLink supplementary files. Start by opening the data file in your computer mounted with SPSS statistical software version 29.

For Cox regression click in the SPSS Menu:

Analyze....Survival....Cox Regression....time: enter time to event....status: enter event yes or no (1 or 0)....Define Event: enter 1....Covariates....click Categorical....Categorical Covariates: enter covariate....click Continue....click Plots....mark Survival....mark Hazard....click Continue....click OK.

For Accelerated failure times models click:

Analyze....Survival....Parametric Accelerated Failure Times (AFT) Models.... mark Survival....enter: "time" or "follow up months" or "timetoevent"....status: enter event....click Define Event...default values are given: Failure/Event = 1, Right Censoring = 0, Left Censoring and Interval Censoring are not defined.... click Continue....Covariate(s) enter treatment, age, gender, etc.....click Model: mark Distribution of Survival Time....mark Weibull....click Continue.... click OK.

In the output sheets several tables of the goodness of fit and p-values of statistical significance of various covariates are included.

4.4 Cox Regression

With Cox regression hazards and hazard ratios are computed (see also the Chap. 2). Also, the Akaike Information Criterion (AIC) is computed. It is an important estimator of the the goodness of fit of a statistical analytic model. The smaller the AIC value the better the goodness of fit of the data. More information of the AICs (Akaike Information Criteria) as measure for goodness of fit of the analytical model is in the Chap. 2 and many subsequent Chaps. With Cox regression AIC is not computed by SPSS statistical software. But it can be easily computed using the omnibus tests of coefficients as shown underneath for the data from our data example. The treatment modality was a significant predictor of survival at p = 0,004, in the Cox regression.

Omnibus Tests of Model Coefficients

-2 Log Likelihood
291,232

Omnibus Tests of Model Coefficients[a]

-2 Log Likelihood	Overall (score)			Change From Previous Step			Change From Previous Block		
	Chi-square	df	Sig.	Chi-square	df	Sig.	Chi-square	df	Sig.
283,059	8,737	1	,003	8,173	1	,004	8,173	1	,004

a. Beginning Block Number 1. Method = Enter

AIC (Akaike Information Criterion) value = 283,059 + kp (=1df (degree of freedom) × the constant "2") = 283,061.

Variables in the Equation

	B	SE	Wald	df	Sig.	Exp(B)
treat	-,930	,325	8,206	1	,004	,394

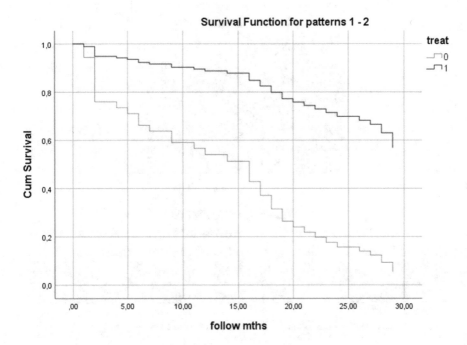

Also, a Kaplan-Meier curve of the data is produced.

4.5   Accelerated Failure Time with Weibull Distribution

The output sheets additionally provide the results from the Weibull Accelerated failure time model.

Model Summary

Data Format	Nonrecurrent
Survival Time	timetoevent
Model	Accelerated failure time (AFT)
Model Distribution	Weibull
Feature Selection	None
Status	event
ADMM	Fast
Estimation Method	Automatically determined by the procedure

Model Fit Statistics

Log Likelihood	-78,805
-2 Log Likelihood	157,611
Akaike's Information Criterion (AIC)	163,611
Hurvich and Tsai's Criterion (AICC)	164,039
Schwarz's Bayesian Criterion (BIC)	169,894

AFT Model Regression Parameters

Parameter	Coefficient	Std. Error	Chi-Squared[a]	Sig.	95% Confidence Interval		Exp. Coefficient	Exp. 95% Confidence Interval	
					Lower	Upper		Lower	Upper
Intercept	2,822	,185	231,887	<,001	2,459	3,186	16,817	11,694	24,182
treat	,855	,285	8,983	,003	,296	1,415	2,352	1,344	4,115
(Scale)[b]	,863	,117	.	.	,662	1,127	.	.	.

a. Degrees of freedom = 1

b. Chi-squared statistic, p-value, and the exponential statistics are not estimated for the scale parameter.

4.6 Accelerated Failure Time Model with Exponential Distribution

The output sheets also provide the results from the Exponential Accelerated failure time model.

Model Summary

Data Format	Nonrecurrent
Survival Time	timetoevent
Model	Accelerated failure time (AFT)
Model Distribution	Exponential
Feature Selection	None
Status	event
ADMM	Fast
Estimation Method	Automatically determined by the procedure

Model Fit Statistics

Log Likelihood	-79,358
-2 Log Likelihood	158,716
Akaike's Information Criterion (AIC)	162,716
Hurvich and Tsai's Criterion (AICC)	162,927
Schwarz's Bayesian Criterion (BIC)	166,905

AFT Model Regression Parameters

Parameter	Coefficient	Std. Error	Chi-Squared[a]	Sig.	95% Confidence Interval		Exp. Coefficient	Exp. 95% Confidence Interval	
					Lower	Upper		Lower	Upper
Intercept	2,803	,213	172,894	<,001	2,385	3,221	16,500	10,864	25,059
treat	,941	,318	8,764	,003	,318	1,564	2,562	1,374	4,777
(Scale)[b]	1,000	.	.	.	.	.	.	.	.

a. Degrees of freedom = 1

b. Scale parameter is fixed at 1 for exponential distribution. Its related statistics are not estimated.

4.7   Accelerated Failure Time Model with Log Normal Distribution

Also, the output sheets additionally provide the results from the log normal Accelerated failure time model.

Model Summary

Data Format	Nonrecurrent
Survival Time	timetoevent
Model	Accelerated failure time (AFT)
Model Distribution	Log-normal
Feature Selection	None
Status	event
ADMM	Fast
Estimation Method	Automatically determined by the procedure

Model Fit Statistics

Log Likelihood	-74,944
-2 Log Likelihood	149,889
Akaike's Information Criterion (AIC)	155,889
Hurvich and Tsai's Criterion (AICC)	156,317
Schwarz's Bayesian Criterion (BIC)	162,172

AFT Model Regression Parameters

| Parameter | Coefficient | Std. Error | Chi-Squared[a] | Sig. | 95% Confidence Interval | | Exp. Coefficient | Exp. 95% Confidence Interval | |
					Lower	Upper		Lower	Upper
Intercept	2,122	,202	110,437	<,001	1,726	2,518	8,349	5,620	12,404
treat	1,463	,293	24,947	<,001	,889	2,037	4,317	2,432	7,665
(Scale)[b]	1,063	,125	.	.	,844	1,340	.	.	.

a. Degrees of freedom = 1

b. Chi-squared statistic, p-value, and the exponential statistics are not estimated for the scale parameter.

4.8   Accelerated Failure Time Model with Log Logistic Distribution

Finally, the output sheets additionally provide the results from the log logistic Accelerated failure time model.

Model Summary

Data Format	Nonrecurrent
Survival Time	timetoevent
Model	Accelerated failure time (AFT)
Model Distribution	Log-logistic
Feature Selection	None
Status	event
ADMM	Fast
Estimation Method	Automatically determined by the procedure

Model Fit Statistics

Log Likelihood	-75,028
-2 Log Likelihood	150,056
Akaike's Information Criterion (AIC)	156,056
Hurvich and Tsai's Criterion (AICC)	156,485
Schwarz's Bayesian Criterion (BIC)	162,339

AFT Model Regression Parameters

Parameter	Coefficient	Std. Error	Chi-Squared[a]	Sig.	95% Confidence Interval		Exp. Coefficient	Exp. 95% Confidence Interval	
					Lower	Upper		Lower	Upper
Intercept	2,101	,220	91,215	<,001	1,670	2,532	8,174	5,311	12,580
treat	1,393	,288	23,353	<,001	,828	1,958	4,028	2,289	7,088
(Scale)[b]	,609	,082	.	.	,468	,793	.	.	.

a. Degrees of freedom = 1

b. Chi-squared statistic, p-value, and the exponential statistics are not estimated for the scale parameter.

4.9   Conclusion

The goodness of fit of the Cox and Accelerated failure time (AFT) models as estimated with the Akaike Information Criterion are summarized underneath.

1. Cox   291,236
2. AFT Weibull   163,611
3. AFT Exponential   162,716
4. AFT Log normal   155,889
5. AFT Log logistics   156,056

The significance of difference between one treatment and the other as estimated with p-values <0,05 are underneath.

1. Cox   0,004
2. AFT Weibull   0,003
3. AFT Exponential   0,003
4. AFT Log normal   0,001
5. AFT Log logistics   0,001

In 60 patients with cardiovascular disease the treatment modality was a significant predictor of event with a p-value of 0,004 in the Cox regression. With the Accelerated failure time model the p-value even fell to $p = 0,001$.

In this parallel group study, the effect of two treatment modalities on survival was assessed. The accelerated failure time (AFT) models performed consistently better than did the Cox regression analysis. However, as the Cox p-value was already very significant, the outcome benefit was limited. With borderline significant Cox results the benefit would probably have been much more spectacular.

References

Five textbooks complementary to the current production and written by the same authors are
(1) Statistics applied to clinical studies 5th edition, 2012,
(2) Machine learning in medicine a complete overview, 2020,
(3) Regression Analysis in Medical Research, 2nd Edition, 2021,
(4) Quantile regression in Clinical Research, 2021,
(5) Kernel Ridge Regression in Clinical research, 2022,
all of them edited by Springer Heidelberg Germany.

Chapter 5
Simple Dataset with Death as Outcome and Treatment Modality, Cholesterol, and Age as Predictors

Abstract In this multiple variables predictive model the effect of three predictors on mortality were assessed. The treatment modality and cholesterol were independend predictors both with p-values of 0,001 in the Cox regression. With the Accelerated failure time model with Weibull distribution equal p-values were obtained.

5.1 Introduction

In a 60 patient parallel group study the effects of (1) treatment modalities, (2) age, and (3) cholesterol on survival will be assessed in a multiple variables predictive model. Survival will be measured in the form of either a hazard, which is the ratio of deaths and non deaths in a random sample, or as a risk which is the proportion of deaths in the same sample. In this chapter hazard and risk will be computed using respectively multiple variables Cox regression and multiple variables Accelerated failure time models.

5.2 Data Example

time to event	event 1 = yes	treat 0 or 1	age years	gender 0 = fem	LDL cholesterol
1,00	1	0	65,00	,00	2,00
1,00	1	0	66,00	,00	2,00
2,00	1	0	73,00	,00	2,00
2,00	1	0	54,00	,00	2,00

(continued)

Supplementary Information The online version contains supplementary material available at https://doi.org/10.1007/978-3-031-31632-6_5.

37

T. J. Cleophas, A. H. Zwinderman, *Modern Survival Analysis in Clinical Research*, https://doi.org/10.1007/978-3-031-31632-6_5

time to event	event 1 = yes	treat 0 or 1	age years	gender 0 = fem	LDL cholesterol
2,00	1	0	46,00	,00	2,00
2,00	1	0	37,00	,00	2,00
2,00	1	0	54,00	,00	2,00
2,00	1	0	66,00	,00	2,00
2,00	1	0	44,00	,00	2,00
3,00	0	0	62,00	,00	2,00
4,00	1	0	57,00	,00	2,00
5,00	1	0	43,00	,00	2,00
6,00	1	0	85,00	,00	2,00
6,00	1	0	46,00	,00	2,00
7,00	1	0	76,00	,00	2,00
9,00	1	0	76,00	,00	2,00
9,00	1	0	65,00	,00	1,00
11,00	1	0	54,00	,00	1,00
12,00	1	0	34,00	,00	1,00
14,00	1	0	45,00	,00	1,00
16,00	1	0	56,00	1,00	1,00
17,00	1	0	67,00	1,00	1,00
18,00	1	0	86,00	1,00	2,00
30,00	0	0	75,00	1,00	2,00
30,00	0	0	65,00	1,00	2,00
30,00	0	0	54,00	1,00	2,00
30,00	0	0	46,00	1,00	2,00
30,00	0	0	54,00	1,00	2,00
30,00	0	0	75,00	1,00	2,00
30,00	0	0	56,00	1,00	2,00
30,00	0	1	56,00	1,00	2,00
30,00	0	1	53,00	1,00	2,00
30,00	0	1	34,00	1,00	2,00
30,00	0	1	35,00	1,00	2,00
30,00	0	1	37,00	1,00	2,00
30,00	0	1	65,00	1,00	2,00
30,00	0	1	45,00	1,00	2,00
30,00	0	1	66,00	1,00	2,00
30,00	0	1	55,00	1,00	2,00
30,00	0	1	88,00	1,00	1,00
29,00	1	1	67,00	1,00	1,00
29,00	1	1	56,00	1,00	1,00
29,00	1	1	54,00	1,00	1,00
28,00	0	1	57,00	1,00	1,00
28,00	1	1	57,00	1,00	1,00
28,00	1	1	76,00	1,00	1,00

(continued)

time to event	event 1 = yes	treat 0 or 1	age years	gender 0 = fem	LDL cholesterol
27,00	1	1	67,00	1,00	1,00
26,00	1	1	66,00	1,00	1,00
24,00	1	1	56,00	1,00	1,00
23,00	1	1	66,00	1,00	1,00
22,00	1	1	84,00	1,00	1,00
22,00	0	1	56,00	1,00	1,00
21,00	1	1	46,00	1,00	1,00
20,00	1	1	45,00	1,00	1,00
19,00	1	1	76,00	1,00	1,00
19,00	1	1	65,00	1,00	1,00
18,00	1	1	45,00	1,00	1,00
17,00	1	1	76,00	1,00	1,00
16,00	1	1	56,00	1,00	1,00
16,00	1	1	45,00	1,00	1,00

5.3   Data Analysis in SPSS Statistical Software Version 29

The commands for Cox regression and for Accelerated failure time models are summarized underneath.

For convenience the data file entitled "Chapter…,……" is in SpringerLink supplementary files. Start by opening the data file in your computer mounted with SPSS statistical software version 29.

For Cox regression click in the SPSS Menu:

Analyze….Survival….Cox Regression….time: enter time to event….status: enter event yes or no (1 or 0)….Define Event: enter 1….Covariates….click Categorical….Categorical Covariates: enter covariate….click Continue….click Plots….mark Survival….mark Hazard….click Continue….click OK.

For Accelerated failure times models click:

Analyze….Survival….Parametric Accelerated Failure Times (AFT) Models…. mark Survival….enter: "time" or "follow up mths" or "timetoevent"….status: enter event….click Define Event…default values are given: Failure/Event = 1, Right Censoring = 0, Left Censoring and Interval Censoring are not defined…. click Continue….Covariate(s) enter treatment, age, gender, etc.….click Model: mark Distribution of Survival Time….mark Weibull….click Continue…. click OK.

In the output sheets several tables of the goodness of fit and p-values of statistical significance of various covariates are included.

5.4   Three Predictors Cox Regression

With Cox regression hazards and hazard ratios are computed (see also the Chap. 2). Also the Akaike Information Criterion (AIC) is computed. It is an important estimator of the the goodness of fit of a statistical analytic model. The smaller the AIC value the better the goodness of fit of the data. More information of the AICs (Akaike Information Criteria) as measure for goodness of fit of the analytical model is in the Chap. 2 and many subsequent Chaps. With Cox regression AIC is not computed by SPSS statistical software. But it can be easily computed using the omnibus tests of coefficients as shown underneath for the data from our data example. Furthermore both treatment modality and elevated cholesterol were significant predictors on mortality at p = 0,001.

Omnibus Tests of Model Coefficients[a]

-2 Log Likelihood	Overall (score)			Change From Previous Step			Change From Previous Block		
	Chi-square	df	Sig.	Chi-square	df	Sig.	Chi-square	df	Sig.
270,666	20,118	3	<,001	20,566	3	<,001	20,566	3	<,001

a. Beginning Block Number 1. Method = Enter

AIC (Akaike Information Criterion) value = 270,666 + kp (=3df (degrees of freedom) × the constant "2") = 270,672.

Variables in the Equation

	B	SE	Wald	df	Sig.	Exp(B)
treat	-1,639	,393	17,362	1	<,001	,194
age	,000	,013	,000	1	,993	1,000
elevated cholesterol	-1,375	,401	11,759	1	<,001	,253

5.5   Three Predictors Accelerated Failure Time (AFT) with Weibull Distribution

The output sheets provide the results from Weibull's AFT model analysis of this multiple variables dataset.

Model Summary

Data Format	Nonrecurrent
Survival Time	timetoevent
Model	Accelerated failure time (AFT)
Model Distribution	Weibull
Feature Selection	None
Status	event
ADMM	Fast
Estimation Method	Automatically determined by the procedure

Model Fit Statistics

Log Likelihood	-74,666
-2 Log Likelihood	149,332
Akaike's Information Criterion (AIC)	159,332
Hurvich and Tsai's Criterion (AICC)	160,444
Schwarz's Bayesian Criterion (BIC)	169,804

AFT Model Regression Parameters

Parameter	Coefficient	Std. Error	Chi-Squared[a]	Sig.	95% Confidence Interval		Exp. Coefficient	Exp. 95% Confidence Interval	
					Lower	Upper		Lower	Upper
Intercept	1,464	,750	3,813	,051	-,006	2,933	4,323	,994	18,791
treat	1,185	,301	15,476	<,001	,595	1,775	3,270	1,812	5,901
age	-,001	,010	,007	,931	-,020	,019	,999	,980	1,019
cholesterol	,835	,294	8,053	,005	,258	1,412	2,306	1,295	4,105
(Scale)[b]	,806	,113			,612	1,062			

a. Degrees of freedom = 1

b. Chi-squared statistic, p-value, and the exponential statistics are not estimated for the scale parameter.

5.6 Three Predictors Accelerated Failure Time Model with Exponential Distribution

The output sheets provide the results from the Exponential AFT model analysis of this multiple variables dataset.

Model Summary

Data Format	Nonrecurrent
Survival Time	timetoevent
Model	Accelerated failure time (AFT)
Model Distribution	Exponential
Feature Selection	None
Status	event
ADMM	Fast
Estimation Method	Automatically determined by the procedure

Model Fit Statistics

Log Likelihood	-75,753
-2 Log Likelihood	151,506
Akaike's Information Criterion (AIC)	159,506
Hurvich and Tsai's Criterion (AICC)	160,234
Schwarz's Bayesian Criterion (BIC)	167,884

AFT Model Regression Parameters

Parameter	Coefficient	Std. Error	Chi-Squared[a]	Sig.	95% Confidence Interval		Exp. Coefficient	Exp. 95% Confidence Interval	
					Lower	Upper		Lower	Upper
Intercept	1,309	,915	2,047	,153	-,484	3,103	3,704	,616	22,267
treat	1,350	,351	14,782	<,001	,662	2,039	3,859	1,939	7,682
age	-,002	,012	,021	,884	-,026	,022	,998	,975	1,022
cholesterol	,947	,356	7,065	,008	,249	1,645	2,578	1,282	5,183
(Scale)[b]	1,000	.	.	.	.	.	.	.	.

a. Degrees of freedom = 1

b. Scale parameter is fixed at 1 for exponential distribution. Its related statistics are not estimated.

5.7   Three Predictors Accelerated Failure Time with Log Normal Distribution

The output sheets provide the results from the log normal AFT model analysis of this multiple variables dataset.

Model Summary

Data Format	Nonrecurrent
Survival Time	timetoevent
Model	Accelerated failure time (AFT)
Model Distribution	Log-normal
Feature Selection	None
Status	event
ADMM	Fast
Estimation Method	Automatically determined by the procedure

Model Fit Statistics

Log Likelihood	-74,114
-2 Log Likelihood	148,228
Akaike's Information Criterion (AIC)	158,228
Hurvich and Tsai's Criterion (AICC)	159,339
Schwarz's Bayesian Criterion (BIC)	168,700

AFT Model Regression Parameters

Parameter	Coefficient	Std. Error	Chi-Squared[a]	Sig.	95% Confidence Interval		Exp. Coefficient	Exp. 95% Confidence Interval	
					Lower	Upper		Lower	Upper
Intercept	1,199	,985	1,482	,223	-,731	3,129	3,316	,481	22,845
treat	1,744	,381	20,929	<,001	,997	2,491	5,720	2,710	12,075
age	,001	,011	,013	,909	-,021	,023	1,001	,980	1,023
cholesterol	,476	,384	1,537	,215	-,277	1,229	1,610	,758	3,419
(Scale)[b]	1,079	,129	.	.	,854	1,365	.	.	.

a. Degrees of freedom = 1
b. Chi-squared statistic, p-value, and the exponential statistics are not estimated for the scale parameter.

5.8   Three Predictors Accelerated Failure Time with Log Logistic Distribution

The output sheets provide the results from the log logistic AFT model analysis of this multiple variables dataset.

Model Summary

Data Format	Nonrecurrent
Survival Time	timetoevent
Model	Accelerated failure time (AFT)
Model Distribution	Log-logistic
Feature Selection	None
Status	event
ADMM	Fast
Estimation Method	Automatically determined by the procedure

Model Fit Statistics

Log Likelihood	-74,380
-2 Log Likelihood	148,760
Akaike's Information Criterion (AIC)	158,760
Hurvich and Tsai's Criterion (AICC)	159,871
Schwarz's Bayesian Criterion (BIC)	169,232

AFT Model Regression Parameters

Parameter	Coefficient	Std. Error	Chi-Squared[a]	Sig.	95% Confidence Interval		Exp. Coefficient	Exp. 95% Confidence Interval	
					Lower	Upper		Lower	Upper
Intercept	1,373	,925	2,201	,138	-,441	3,187	3,947	,643	24,213
treat	1,585	,354	20,027	<,001	,891	2,280	4,881	2,438	9,774
age	,001	,011	,015	,904	-,019	,022	1,001	,981	1,022
cholesterol	,388	,355	1,192	,275	-,308	1,085	1,474	,735	2,958
(Scale)[b]	,616	,084	.	.	,472	,805	.	.	.

a. Degrees of freedom = 1

b. Chi-squared statistic, p-value, and the exponential statistics are not estimated for the scale parameter.

5.9   Conclusion

	Akaike information criterion	p-value of significance of covariances used as predictors		
		treatment	age	cholesterol
Cox	270,666 + 3 × 2 (270,672)	<0,001	0,993	<0,001

AFT (accelerated failure time) models	Akaike information	treatment	age	cholesterol
Weibull	159,332	<0,001	0,931	<0,001
Exponential	159,506	<,0001	0,884	0,008
Log normal	158,228	<0,001	0,909	0,215
Log logistics	158,760	<0,001	0,904	0,275

The goodness of fit values as measured with AICs (Akaike Information Criteria) of the Cox regression was much worse than those of the AFT models. More explanations of AICs are in the Chap. 3.

The p-values of the AFT models of Weibull and Exponential were similarly sized to those of the Cox regression. The AFT p-values of the predictor cholesterol, however, were not statistically significant with the log normal and log logistics distributions.

References

Five textbooks complementary to the current production and written by the same authors are
(1) Statistics applied to clinical studies 5th edition, 2012,
(2) Machine learning in medicine a complete overview, 2020,
(3) Regression Analysis in Medical Research, 2nd Edition, 2021,
(4) Quantile regression in Clinical Research, 2021,
(5) Kernel Ridge Regression in Clinical research, 2022,
all of them edited by Springer Heidelberg Germany.

Chapter 6
Glioma Brain Cancer

Abstract In 29 patients with glioma brain cancer treatment modality was an insignificant predictor of event with a p-value of 0,083. With the Accelerated failure time model with exponential distribution the p-value fell to 0,047, and became thus statistically significant at p < 0,05.

6.1 Introduction

Medical treatments may influence survival. However, documented proof is often missing. In this chapter the effect on survival of a novel treatment is assessed against a control treatment. Survival can be measured in the form of either a hazard, which is the ratio of deaths and non-deaths in a random sample, or as a risk which is the proportion of deaths in the same sample. In this chapter hazard and risk of the same data will be computed in a 29 patient parallel group study using respectively Cox regression and Accelerated failure time models.

6.2 Data Example

The dataset is from www.healthline.com>health>brain-tumor, December 1, 2022. The effect of two treatment modalities on survival time (days) was assessed with Cox regression and Accelerated Failure Time models.

Supplementary Information The online version contains supplementary material available at https://doi.org/10.1007/978-3-031-31632-6_6.

T. J. Cleophas, A. H. Zwinderman, *Modern Survival Analysis in Clinical Research*, https://doi.org/10.1007/978-3-031-31632-6_6

Time to survival	event	treatment
10,000	1,00	1,00
18,000	1,00	1,00
25,000	1,00	1,00
83,000	1,00	1,00
210,000	1,00	1,00
225,000	1,00	1,00
248,000	1,00	1,00
270,000	1,00	1,00
370,000	1,00	1,00
490,000	1,00	1,00
599,000	,00	1,00
700,000	1,00	1,00
740,000	1,00	1,00
740,000	,00	1,00
20,000	1,00	2,00
80,000	,00	2,00
120,000	1,00	2,00
125,000	1,00	2,00
200,000	,00	2,00
265,000	1,00	2,00
375,000	1,00	2,00
365,000	1,00	2,00
490,000	1,00	2,00
600,000	,00	2,00
800,000	,00	2,00
805,000	,00	2,00
900,000	,00	2,00
950,000	,00	2,00
1000,000	,00	2,00

6.3   Data Analysis in SPSS Statistical Software Version 29

The commands for Cox regression and for Accelerated failure time models are summarized underneath.

For convenience the data file entitled "Chapter 6,……" is in SpringerLink supplementary files. Start by opening the data file in your computer mounted with SPSS statistical software version 29.

For Cox regression click in the SPSS Menu:

Analyze….Survival….Cox Regression….time: enter time to event….status: enter
event yes or no (1 or 0)….Define Event: enter 1….Covariates….click
Categorical….Categorical Covariates: enter covariate….click Continue….click
Plots….mark Survival….mark Hazard….click Continue….click OK.

For Accelerated failure times models click:

Analyze….Survival….Parametric Accelerated Failure Times (AFT) Models….mark
Survival….enter: "time" or "follow up mths" or "timetoevent"….status: enter
event….click Define Event…default values are given: Failure/Event = 1, Right
Censoring = 0, Left Censoring and Interval Censoring are not defined….click
Continue….Covariate(s) enter treatment, age, gender, etc….click Model: mark
Distribution of Survival Time….mark Weibull….click Continue….click OK.

In the output sheets several tables of the goodness of fit and p-values of statistical
significance of various covariates are included.

6.4 Cox Regression

Using the commands from the above Sect. 6.3 the computer will provide in the
output sheets the underneath tables. The treatment modality is a significant predictor of survival at $p = 0,083$.

Omnibus Tests of Model Coefficients[a]

-2 Log Likelihood	Overall (score)			Change From Previous Step			Change From Previous Block		
	Chi-square	df	Sig.	Chi-square	df	Sig.	Chi-square	df	Sig.
104,866	3,169	1	,075	3,137	1	,077	3,137	1	,077

a. Beginning Block Number 1. Method = Enter

Variables in the Equation

	B	SE	Wald	df	Sig.	Exp(B)
treat	-,827	,478	2,999	1	,083	,437

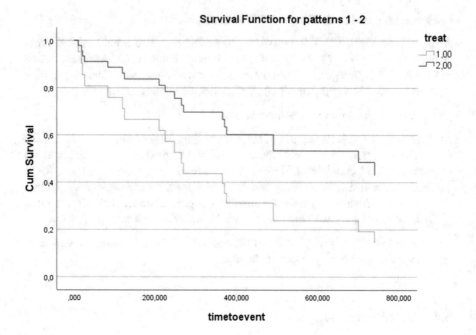

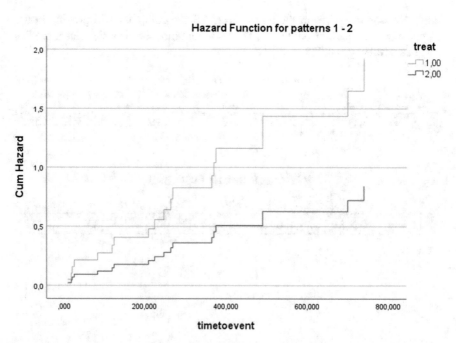

6.5   Accelerated Failure Time (AFT) Model with Weibull Distribution

The output sheets provide the results from Weibull's AFT analysis.

Model Summary

Data Format	Nonrecurrent
Survival Time	timetoevent
Model	Accelerated failure time (AFT)
Model Distribution	Weibull
Feature Selection	None
Status	event
ADMM	Fast
Estimation Method	Automatically determined by the procedure

Model Fit Statistics

Log Likelihood	-42,715
-2 Log Likelihood	85,431
Akaike's Information Criterion (AIC)	91,431
Hurvich and Tsai's Criterion (AICC)	92,391
Schwarz's Bayesian Criterion (BIC)	95,533

AFT Model Regression Parameters

Parameter	Coefficient	Std. Error	Chi-Squared[a]	Sig.	95% Confidence Interval		Exp. Coefficient	Exp. 95% Confidence Interval	
					Lower	Upper		Lower	Upper
Intercept	4,904	,817	36,066	<,001	3,303	6,504	134,797	27,204	667,918
treat	1,047	,569	3,386	,066	-,068	2,163	2,850	,934	8,698
(Scale)[b]	1,152	,229	.	.	,779	1,702	.	.	.

a. Degrees of freedom = 1

b. Chi-squared statistic, p-value, and the exponential statistics are not estimated for the scale parameter.

6.6   The Accelerated Failure Time (AFT) with Exponential Distribution

The output sheets provide the results from the exponential AFT model.

Model Summary

Data Format	Nonrecurrent
Survival Time	timetoevent
Model	Accelerated failure time (AFT)
Model Distribution	Exponential
Feature Selection	None
Status	event
ADMM	Fast
Estimation Method	Automatically determined by the procedure

Model Fit Statistics

Log Likelihood	-42,981
-2 Log Likelihood	85,962
Akaike's Information Criterion (AIC)	89,962
Hurvich and Tsai's Criterion (AICC)	90,424
Schwarz's Bayesian Criterion (BIC)	92,697

AFT Model Regression Parameters

Parameter	Coefficient	Std. Error	Chi-Squared[a]	Sig.	95% Confidence Interval		Exp. Coefficient	Exp. 95% Confidence Interval	
					Lower	Upper		Lower	Upper
Intercept	5,031	,690	53,163	<,001	3,679	6,384	153,154	39,605	592,262
treat	,945	,476	3,947	,047	,013	1,877	2,573	1,013	6,534
(Scale)[b]	1,000								

a. Degrees of freedom = 1

b. Scale parameter is fixed at 1 for exponential distribution. Its related statistics are not estimated.

6.7   Accelerated Failure Time (AFT) with Log Normal Distribution

The output sheets provide the results from the log normal AFT model.

Model Summary

Data Format	Nonrecurrent
Survival Time	timetoevent
Model	Accelerated failure time (AFT)
Model Distribution	Log-normal
Feature Selection	None
Status	event
ADMM	Fast
Estimation Method	Automatically determined by the procedure

Model Fit Statistics

Log Likelihood	-43,212
-2 Log Likelihood	86,425
Akaike's Information Criterion (AIC)	92,425
Hurvich and Tsai's Criterion (AICC)	93,385
Schwarz's Bayesian Criterion (BIC)	96,527

AFT Model Regression Parameters

Parameter	Coefficient	Std. Error	Chi-Squared[a]	Sig.	95% Confidence Interval		Exp. Coefficient	Exp. 95% Confidence Interval	
					Lower	Upper		Lower	Upper
Intercept	4,170	1,008	17,119	<,001	2,195	6,146	64,726	8,978	466,649
treat	1,179	,659	3,198	,074	-,113	2,472	3,252	,893	11,841
(Scale)[b]	1,627	,278	.	.	1,164	2,273	.	.	.

a. Degrees of freedom = 1

b. Chi-squared statistic, p-value, and the exponential statistics are not estimated for the scale parameter.

6.8   Accelerated Failure Time with Log-logistic Distribution

The output sheets provide the results from the log logistic AFT model.

Model Summary

Data Format	Nonrecurrent
Survival Time	timetoevent
Model	Accelerated failure time (AFT)
Model Distribution	Log-logistic
Feature Selection	None
Status	event
ADMM	Fast
Estimation Method	Automatically determined by the procedure

Model Fit Statistics

Log Likelihood	-43,378
-2 Log Likelihood	86,757
Akaike's Information Criterion (AIC)	92,757
Hurvich and Tsai's Criterion (AICC)	93,717
Schwarz's Bayesian Criterion (BIC)	96,859

AFT Model Regression Parameters

Parameter	Coefficient	Std. Error	Chi-Squared[a]	Sig.	95% Confidence Interval		Exp. Coefficient	Exp. 95% Confidence Interval	
					Lower	Upper		Lower	Upper
Intercept	4,431	,990	20,030	<,001	2,491	6,372	84,057	12,071	585,350
treat	1,039	,646	2,590	,108	-,226	2,305	2,828	,797	10,027
(Scale)[b]	,934	,182	.	.	,637	1,368	.	.	.

a. Degrees of freedom = 1

b. Chi-squared statistic, p-value, and the exponential statistics are not estimated for the scale parameter.

6.9   Conclusion

Out of four AFT models the best power was provided by the Exponential AFT model with an AIC (Akaike Information Criterion) value of 89,962, and a p-value of difference between the two treatments of p = 0,047.

	AIC value	p-value of significant difference from zero
Cox	104,868	0,083
AFT Weibull	91,431	0,066
AFT Exponential	89,962	0,047
AFT Log normal	92,425	0,074
AFT Log logistics	92,757	0,108

References

Five textbooks complementary to the current production and written by the same authors are
(1) Statistics applied to clinical studies 5th edition, 2012,
(2) Machine learning in medicine a complete overview, 2020,
(3) Regression Analysis in Medical Research, 2nd Edition, 2021,
(4) Quantile regression in Clinical Research, 2021,
(5) Kernel Ridge Regression in Clinical research, 2022,
all of them edited by Springer Heidelberg Germany.

Chapter 7
Linoleic Acid for Colonic Carcinoma

Abstract In 28 patients with metastatic colonic cancer the treatment modality was a significant predictor of event with a p-value of 0,010 in the Cox regression. With the Accelerated failure time models the best predictive p-value was $p = 0,001$ which was ten times better than that of the Cox model. For all of the AFT (Accelerated failure time) models the AIC (Akaike Information Criterion) goodness of fit measure was over twice better with AIC values around 25,000 as compared to that of the Cox regression of close to 70,000 (the smaller the value, the better the fit). AFT p-values were correspondingly generally much smaller than those of the Cox regression.

7.1 Introduction

The effect on survival of treatment with linoleic acid or placebo in 28 patients with metastatic colonic carcinoma will be tested with Cox regression versus accelerated failure time modeling. "Stop study without event" means, that the patient's time in the study is included but the count for event is zero. The patient is classified to be censored.

7.2 Data Example

Time to event (months)	group	event (1,00) or stop study (0,00)
12,00	1,00	,00
12,00	2,00	1,00
13,00	1,00	,00
15,00	1,00	,00
15,00	2,00	1,00

(continued)

Supplementary Information The online version contains supplementary material available at https://doi.org/10.1007/978-3-031-31632-6_7.

57

Time to event (months)	group	event (1,00) or stop study (0,00)
16,00	1,00	,00
16,00	2,00	1,00
18,00	2,00	1,00
18,00	2,00	1,00
20,00	2,00	1,00
20,00	1,00	,00
22,00	2,00	,00
24,00	1,00	1,00
24,00	2,00	1,00
24,00	1,00	,00
27,00	1,00	,00
28,00	2,00	1,00
28,00	2,00	1,00
28,00	2,00	1,00
30,00	2,00	1,00
30,00	2,00	1,00
32,00	1,00	1,00
33,00	2,00	1,00
34,00	1,00	,00
36,00	1,00	,00
36,00	1,00	,00
42,00	2,00	1,00
44,00	1,00	,00

7.3   Data Analysis in SPSS Statistical Software Version 29

The commands for Cox regression and for Accelerated failure time models are summarized underneath.

For convenience the data file entitled "Chapter 7,......" is in SpringerLink supplementary files. Start by opening the data file in your computer mounted with SPSS statistical software version 29.

For Cox regression click in the SPSS Menu:

Analyze....Survival....Cox Regression....time: enter time to event....status: enter event yes or no (1 or 0)....Define Event: enter 1....Covariates....click Categorical....Categorical Covariates: enter covariate....click Continue....click Plots....mark Survival....mark Hazard....click Continue....click OK.

For Accelerated failure times models click:

Analyze....Survival....Parametric Accelerated Failure Times (AFT) Models.... mark Survival....enter: "time" or "follow up mths" or "timetoevent"....status: enter event....click Define Event...default values are given: Failure/Event = 1, Right Censoring = 0, Left Censoring and Interval Censoring are not defined....

click Continue....Covariate(s) enter treatment, age, gender, etc....click Model: mark Distribution of Survival Time....mark Weibull....click Continue.... click OK.

In the output sheets several tables of the goodness of fit and p-values of statistical significance of various covariates are included.

7.4 Cox Regression

Using the commands from the above Sect. 7.3 the computer will provide in the output sheets the underneath tables. The treatment modality is a significant predictor of survival at $p = 0,010$.

Omnibus Tests of Model Coefficients

-2 Log Likelihood
81,090

Omnibus Tests of Model Coefficients[a]

-2 Log Likelihood	Overall (score)			Change From Previous Step			Change From Previous Block		
	Chi-square	df	Sig.	Chi-square	df	Sig.	Chi-square	df	Sig.
70,920	9,010	1	,003	10,170	1	,001	10,170	1	,001

a. Beginning Block Number 1. Method = Enter

Variables in the Equation

	B	SE	Wald	df	Sig.	Exp(B)
group	1,980	,763	6,724	1	,010	7,241

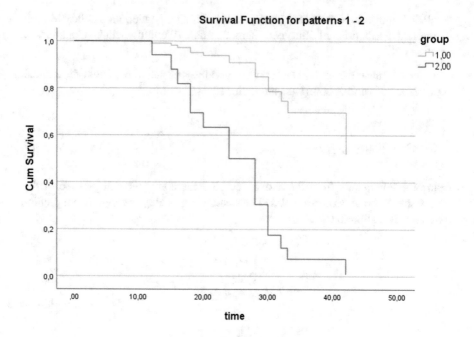

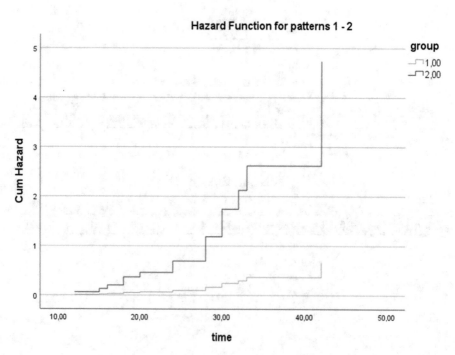

7.5   Accelerated Failure Time (AFT) with Weibull Distribution

The output sheets provide the results of Weibull's AFT analysis.

Model Summary

Data Format	Nonrecurrent
Survival Time	time
Model	Accelerated failure time (AFT)
Model Distribution	Weibull
Feature Selection	None
Status	stopstudy
ADMM	Fast
Estimation Method	Automatically determined by the procedure

Model Fit Statistics

Log Likelihood	-9,124
-2 Log Likelihood	18,249
Akaike's Information Criterion (AIC)	24,249
Hurvich and Tsai's Criterion (AICC)	25,249
Schwarz's Bayesian Criterion (BIC)	28,245

AFT Model Regression Parameters

Parameter	Coefficient	Std. Error	Chi-Squared[a]	Sig.	95% Confidence Interval		Exp. Coefficient	Exp. 95% Confidence Interval	
					Lower	Upper		Lower	Upper
Intercept	4,540	,449	102,472	<,001	3,661	5,420	93,735	38,914	225,785
group	-,610	,238	6,555	,010	-1,077	-,143	,543	,341	,867
(Scale)[b]	,289	,055	.	.	,200	,418	.	.	.

a. Degrees of freedom = 1

b. Chi-squared statistic, p-value, and the exponential statistics are not estimated for the scale parameter.

7.6   Accelerated Failure Time (AFT) with Exponential Distribution

The output sheets provide the results of the exponential AFT analysis.

Model Summary

Data Format	Nonrecurrent
Survival Time	time
Model	Accelerated failure time (AFT)
Model Distribution	Exponential
Feature Selection	None
Status	stopstudy
ADMM	Fast
Estimation Method	Automatically determined by the procedure

Model Fit Statistics

Log Likelihood	-21,246
-2 Log Likelihood	42,493
Akaike's Information Criterion (AIC)	46,493
Hurvich and Tsai's Criterion (AICC)	46,973
Schwarz's Bayesian Criterion (BIC)	49,157

AFT Model Regression Parameters

Parameter	Coefficient	Std. Error	Chi-Squared[a]	Sig.	95% Confidence Interval		Exp. Coefficient	Exp. 95% Confidence Interval	
					Lower	Upper		Lower	Upper
Intercept	6,971	1,439	23,469	<,001	4,151	9,791	1065,251	63,478	17876,303
group	-1,856	,756	6,033	,014	-3,338	-,375	,156	,036	,687
(Scale)[b]	1,000	.	.		.	.	.	.	.

a. Degrees of freedom = 1
b. Scale parameter is fixed at 1 for exponential distribution. Its related statistics are not estimated.

7.7   Accelerated Failure Time (AFT) with Log Normal Distribution

The output sheets provide the results of the log normal AFT analysis.

Model Summary

Data Format	Nonrecurrent
Survival Time	time
Model	Accelerated failure time (AFT)
Model Distribution	Log-normal
Feature Selection	None
Status	stopstudy
ADMM	Fast
Estimation Method	Automatically determined by the procedure

Model Fit Statistics

Log Likelihood	-8,796
-2 Log Likelihood	17,593
Akaike's Information Criterion (AIC)	23,593
Hurvich and Tsai's Criterion (AICC)	24,593
Schwarz's Bayesian Criterion (BIC)	27,589

AFT Model Regression Parameters

Parameter	Coefficient	Std. Error	Chi-Squared[a]	Sig.	95% Confidence Interval		Exp. Coefficient	Exp. 95% Confidence Interval	
					Lower	Upper		Lower	Upper
Intercept	4,371	,349	157,145	<,001	3,688	5,055	79,135	39,954	156,739
group	-,607	,191	10,160	,001	-,981	-,234	,545	,375	,791
(Scale)[b]	,344	,061	.	.	,243	,488	.	.	.

a. Degrees of freedom = 1

b. Chi-squared statistic, p-value, and the exponential statistics are not estimated for the scale parameter.

7.8   Accelerated Failure Time (AFT) with Log Logistic Distribution

He output sheets provide the results of the log logistic AFT analysis.

Model Summary

Data Format	Nonrecurrent
Survival Time	time
Model	Accelerated failure time (AFT)
Model Distribution	Log-logistic
Feature Selection	None
Status	stopstudy
ADMM	Fast
Estimation Method	Automatically determined by the procedure

Model Fit Statistics

Log Likelihood	-9,419
-2 Log Likelihood	18,838
Akaike's Information Criterion (AIC)	24,838
Hurvich and Tsai's Criterion (AICC)	25,838
Schwarz's Bayesian Criterion (BIC)	28,834

AFT Model Regression Parameters

Parameter	Coefficient	Std. Error	Chi-Squared[a]	Sig.	95% Confidence Interval Lower	95% Confidence Interval Upper	Exp. Coefficient	Exp. 95% Confidence Interval Lower	Exp. 95% Confidence Interval Upper
Intercept	4,362	,372	137,643	<,001	3,633	5,090	78,389	37,827	162,447
group	-,595	,203	8,556	,003	-,994	-,196	,552	,370	,822
(Scale)[b]	,204	,041	.	.	,138	,303	.	.	.

a. Degrees of freedom = 1

b. Chi-squared statistic, p-value, and the exponential statistics are not estimated for the scale parameter.

7.9   Conclusion

The best predictive AFT p-value was p = 0,001 which was ten times smaller and thus better than that of the Cox model.

For all of the AFT (Accelerated failure time) models the AIC (Akaike Information Criterion) goodness of fit measure was over twice better with AIC values around 25,000 as compared to that of the Cox regression over 70,000 (the smaller the value, the better the fit). AFT p-values were correspondingly generally smaller than those of the Cox regression.

	Akaike Information Criterion	p-value of difference between two treatments
Cox	70,922	0,010
AFT Weibull	24,249	0,010
AFT Exponential	46,493	0,014
AFT Log normal	23,593	0,001
AFT log logistics	24,838	0,003

Nevertheless, the AFT Weibull model and the Cox regression produced equally significant p-values.

References

Five textbooks complementary to the current production and written by the same authors are
(1) Statistics applied to clinical studies 5th edition, 2012,
(2) Machine learning in medicine a complete overview, 2020,
(3) Regression Analysis in Medical Research, 2nd Edition, 2021,
(4) Quantile regression in Clinical Research, 2021,
(5) Kernel Ridge Regression in Clinical research, 2022,
all of them edited by Springer Heidelberg Germany.

Chapter 8
The Effect on Survival of Maintained Chemotherapy with Acute Myelogenous Leucemia

Abstract In 23 patients with acute myeloid leucemia maintained chemotherapy or discontinued chemotherapy were compared in a parallel group study. Maintenance was an insignificant predictor of survival with a p-value of 0,078. With the Accelerated failure time model with a Weibull distribution the p-value fell to 0,015.

8.1 Introduction

Medical treatments may influence survival. However documented proof is often missing. In this chapter the effect on survival of maintained chemotherapy will be assessed against discontinued treatment as control. Survival can be measured in the form of either a hazard, which is the ratio of deaths and non deaths in a random sample, or as a risk which is the proportion of deaths in the same sample. In this chapter hazard and risk of the same data will be computed in a 23 patient parallel group study using respectively Cox regression and Accelerated failure time models.

8.2 Data Example

A dataset from Miller and Rupert's edition Survival analysis, Wiley & Sons, 1997, ISBN 0-471-25218-2 has been used as example for comparing Cox versus Accelerated Failure Time analysis. 23 Patients were followed for 161 weeks.

Supplementary Information The online version contains supplementary material available at https://doi.org/10.1007/978-3-031-31632-6_8.

Survival weeks	event	patient	group
5,00	1,00	12,00	1,00
5,00	1,00	13,00	1,00
8,00	1,00	14,00	1,00
8,00	1,00	15,00	1,00
9,00	1,00	1,00	2,00
12,00	1,00	16,00	1,00
13,00	1,00	2,00	2,00
13,00	,00	3,00	2,00
16,00	,00	17,00	1,00
18,00	1,00	4,00	2,00
23,00	1,00	5,00	2,00
23,00	1,00	18,00	1,00
27,00	1,00	19,00	1,00
28,00	,00	6,00	2,00
30,00	1,00	20,00	1,00
31,00	1,00	7,00	2,00
33,00	1,00	21,00	1,00
34,00	1,00	8,00	2,00
43,00	1,00	22,00	1,00
45,00	,00	9,00	2,00
45,00	1,00	23,00	1,00
48,00	1,00	10,00	2,00
161,00	,00	11,00	2,00

8.3   Data Analysis in SPSS Statistical Software Version 29

The commands for Cox regression and for Accelerated failure time models are summarized underneath.

For convenience the data file entitled "Chapter 8,......" is in SpringerLink supplementary files. Start by opening the data file in your computer mounted with SPSS statistical software version 29.

For Cox regression click in the SPSS Menu:

Analyze....Survival....Cox Regression....time: enter time to event....status: enter event yes or no (1 or 0)....Define Event: enter 1....Covariates....click Categorical....Categorical Covariates: enter covariate....click Continue....click Plots....mark Survival....mark Hazard....click Continue....click OK.

For Accelerated failure times models click:

Analyze....Survival....Parametric Accelerated Failure Times (AFT) Models.... mark Survival....enter: "time" or "follow up mths" or "timetoevent"....status: enter event....click Define Event...default values are given: Failure/Event = 1,

Right Censoring = 0, Left Censoring and Interval Censoring are not defined.…
click Continue.…Covariate(s) enter treatment, age, gender, etc.…click Model:
mark Distribution of Survival Time.…mark Weibull.…click Continue.…
click OK.

In the output sheets several tables of the goodness of fit and p-values of statistical
significance of various covariates are included.

8.4 Cox Regression

With Cox regression hazards and hazard ratios are computed (see also the Chap. 2).
Also the Akaike Information Criterion (AIC) is computed. It is an important estimator the goodness of fit of a statistical analysis model. The smaller the AIC value the
better the goodness of fit of the data. More information of the AICs (Akaike
Information Criteria) as measure for goodness of fit of the analytical model is in the
Chap. 2 and many subsequent Chaps. With Cox regression AIC is not computed by
SPSS statistical software. But it can be calculated using the omnibus tests of coefficients (see Chap. 4). Using the commands from the above Sect. 8.3 the computer
will provide in the output sheets the underneath tables. The treatment modality is an
insignificant predictor of survival at p = 0,078.

Also Kaplan-Meier graphs are in the output.

Omnibus Tests of Model Coefficients

-2 Log Likelihood
85,796

Omnibus Tests of Model Coefficients[a]

-2 Log Likelihood	Overall (score)			Change From Previous Step			Change From Previous Block		
	Chi-square	df	Sig.	Chi-square	df	Sig.	Chi-square	df	Sig.
82,500	3,323	1	,068	3,296	1	,069	3,296	1	,069

a. Beginning Block Number 1. Method = Enter

Variables in the Equation

	B	SE	Wald	df	Sig.	Exp(B)
group	-,904	,512	3,116	1	,078	,405

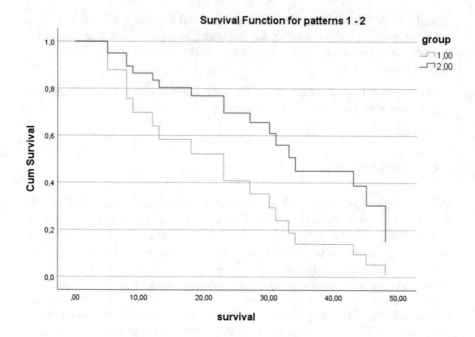

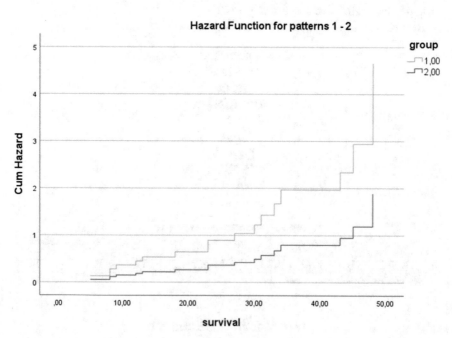

8.5   Accelerated Failure Time (AFT) with Weibull Distribution

The output sheets provide the results of the Weibull AFT analysis.

Model Summary

Data Format	Nonrecurrent
Survival Time	survival
Model	Accelerated failure time (AFT)
Model Distribution	Weibull
Feature Selection	None
Status	event
ADMM	Fast
Estimation Method	Automatically determined by the procedure

Model Fit Statistics

Log Likelihood	-28,142
-2 Log Likelihood	56,285
Akaike's Information Criterion (AIC)	62,285
Hurvich and Tsai's Criterion (AICC)	63,548
Schwarz's Bayesian Criterion (BIC)	65,691

AFT Model Regression Parameters

Parameter	Coefficient	Std. Error	Chi-Squared[a]	Sig.	95% Confidence Interval		Exp. Coefficient	Exp. 95% Confidence Interval	
					Lower	Upper		Lower	Upper
Intercept	2,250	,564	15,905	<,001	1,144	3,356	9,491	3,141	28,685
group	,929	,383	5,903	,015	,180	1,679	2,533	1,197	5,360
(Scale)[b]	,791	,141	.	.	,558	1,122	.	.	.

a. Degrees of freedom = 1
b. Chi-squared statistic, p-value, and the exponential statistics are not estimated for the scale parameter.

8.6   Accelerated Failure Time (AFT) with Exponential Distribution

The output sheets provide the results from the exponential AFT analysis.

Model Summary

Data Format	Nonrecurrent
Survival Time	survival
Model	Accelerated failure time (AFT)
Model Distribution	Exponential
Feature Selection	None
Status	event
ADMM	Fast
Estimation Method	Automatically determined by the procedure

Model Fit Statistics

Log Likelihood	-28,908
-2 Log Likelihood	57,816
Akaike's Information Criterion (AIC)	61,816
Hurvich and Tsai's Criterion (AICC)	62,416
Schwarz's Bayesian Criterion (BIC)	64,087

AFT Model Regression Parameters

Parameter	Coefficient	Std. Error	Chi-Squared[a]	Sig.	95% Confidence Interval		Exp. Coefficient	Exp. 95% Confidence Interval	
					Lower	Upper		Lower	Upper
Intercept	2,185	,712	9,429	,002	,790	3,580	8,893	2,204	35,880
group	,958	,483	3,927	,048	,010	1,906	2,607	1,010	6,724
(Scale)[b]	1,000	.	.				.		

a. Degrees of freedom = 1

b. Scale parameter is fixed at 1 for exponential distribution. Its related statistics are not estimated.

8.7   Accelerated Failure Time (AFT) with Log Normal Distribution

The output sheets provide the results from the log normal AFT analysis.

Model Summary

Data Format	Nonrecurrent
Survival Time	survival
Model	Accelerated failure time (AFT)
Model Distribution	Log-normal
Feature Selection	None
Status	event
ADMM	Fast
Estimation Method	Automatically determined by the procedure

Model Fit Statistics

Log Likelihood	-26,548
-2 Log Likelihood	53,097
Akaike's Information Criterion (AIC)	59,097
Hurvich and Tsai's Criterion (AICC)	60,360
Schwarz's Bayesian Criterion (BIC)	62,503

AFT Model Regression Parameters

Parameter	Coefficient	Std. Error	Chi-Squared[a]	Sig.	95% Confidence Interval		Exp. Coefficient	Exp. 95% Confidence Interval	
					Lower	Upper		Lower	Upper
Intercept	2,130	,581	13,455	<,001	,992	3,268	8,414	2,696	26,260
group	,724	,380	3,629	,057	-,021	1,470	2,064	,979	4,349
(Scale)[b]	,865	,147	.	.	,620	1,205	.	.	.

a. Degrees of freedom = 1

b. Chi-squared statistic, p-value, and the exponential statistics are not estimated for the scale parameter.

8.8   Accelerated Failure Time (AFT) with Log Logistic Distribution

The output sheets provide the results from the AFT log logistic analysis.

Model Summary

Data Format	Nonrecurrent
Survival Time	survival
Model	Accelerated failure time (AFT)
Model Distribution	Log-logistic
Feature Selection	None
Status	event
ADMM	Fast
Estimation Method	Automatically determined by the procedure

Model Fit Statistics

Log Likelihood	-26,974
-2 Log Likelihood	53,947
Akaike's Information Criterion (AIC)	59,947
Hurvich and Tsai's Criterion (AICC)	61,210
Schwarz's Bayesian Criterion (BIC)	63,354

AFT Model Regression Parameters

Parameter	Coefficient	Std. Error	Chi-Squared[a]	Sig.	95% Confidence Interval Lower	95% Confidence Interval Upper	Exp. Coefficient	Exp. 95% Confidence Interval Lower	Exp. 95% Confidence Interval Upper
Intercept	2,294	,608	14,242	<,001	1,103	3,485	9,915	3,012	32,637
group	,604	,393	2,362	,124	-,166	1,375	1,830	,847	3,956
(Scale)[b]	,513	,098	.	.	,353	,747	.	.	.

a. Degrees of freedom = 1

b. Chi-squared statistic, p-value, and the exponential statistics are not estimated for the scale parameter.

8.9 Conclusion

	Akaike Information Criterion	P-value of Difference between Treatments
Cox	82,502	0,078
AFT Weibull	62,285	0,015
AFT Exponential	61,816	0,048
AFT Log normal	59,097	0,057
AFT Log logistics	59,947	0,124

The best fit model for the dataset was the AFT Weibull distribution with a p-value of difference between treatments of 0,015, while the Cox model provided a p-value of only 0,078, and was thus not statistically significant. In this example the AFT results were able to make a difference between no efficacy and a pretty significant efficacy of the new treatment.

References

Five textbooks complementary to the current production and written by the same authors are
(1) Statistics applied to clinical studies 5th edition, 2012,
(2) Machine learning in medicine a complete overview, 2020,
(3) Regression Analysis in Medical Research, 2nd Edition, 2021,
(4) Quantile regression in Clinical Research, 2021,
(5) Kernel Ridge Regression in Clinical research, 2022,
all of them edited by Springer Heidelberg Germany.

Chapter 9
Eighty Four Month Parallel Group Mortality Study

Abstract In a 15 patient mortality study the treatment modality was an insignificant predictor of mortality with a p-value of 0,138. With the Accelerated failure time model with Weibull distribution the p-value fell to 0,008.

9.1 Introduction

Medical treatments may influence survival. However documented proof is often missing. In this chapter the effect on survival of a novel treatment is assessed against a control treatment. Survival can be measured in the form of either a hazard, which is the ratio of deaths and non deaths in a random sample, or as a risk which is the proportion of deaths in the same sample. In this chapter hazard and risk of the same data will be computed in a 15 patient parallel group study using respectively Cox regression and Accelerated failure time models.

9.2 Data Example

In 15 patients with stage 4 non-hodgkin lymphoma a 84 month parallel group mortality study of two treatments was performed. Only one out of 15 patient was censored, because he had no event at the time he left the study.

Supplementary Information The online version contains supplementary material available at https://doi.org/10.1007/978-3-031-31632-6_9.

T. J. Cleophas, A. H. Zwinderman, *Modern Survival Analysis in Clinical Research*, https://doi.org/10.1007/978-3-031-31632-6_9

Months	event	group
10,00	,00	1,00
10,00	1,00	1,00
14,00	1,00	1,00
15,00	1,00	1,00
16,00	1,00	1,00
17,00	1,00	1,00
18,00	1,00	1,00
21,00	1,00	1,00
34,00	1,00	1,00
14,00	1,00	2,00
20,00	1,00	2,00
23,00	1,00	2,00
25,00	1,00	2,00
27,00	1,00	2,00
84,00	1,00	2,00

9.3   Data Analysis in SPSS Statistical Software Version 29

The commands for Cox regression and for Accelerated failure time models are sum-marized underneath.

For convenience the data file entitled "Chapter 9,..." is in SpringerLink supple-mentary files. Start by opening the data file in your computer mounted with SPSS statistical software version 29.

For Cox regression click in the SPSS Menu:

Analyze....Survival....Cox Regression....time: enter time to event....status: enter event yes or no (1 or 0)....Define Event: enter 1....Covariates....click Categorical....Categorical Covariates: enter covariate....click Continue....click Plots....mark Survival....mark Hazard....click Continue....click OK.

For Accelerated failure times models click:

Analyze....Survival....Parametric Accelerated Failure Times (AFT) Models.... mark Survival....enter: "time" or "follow up mths" or "timetoevent"....status: enter event....click Define Event...default values are given: Failure/Event = 1, Right Censoring = 0, Left Censoring and Interval Censoring are not defined.... click Continue....Covariate(s) enter treatment, age, gender, etc....click Model: mark Distribution of Survival Time....mark Weibull....click Continue.... click OK.

In the output sheets several tables of the goodness of fit and p-values of statistical significance of various covariates are included.

9.4 Cox Regression

With Cox regression hazards and hazard ratios are computed (see also the Chap. 2). Also the Akaike Information Criterion (AIC) is computed. It is an important estimator the goodness of fit of a statistical analysis model. The smaller the AIC value the better the goodness of fit of the data. More information of the AICs (Akaike Information Criteria) as measure for goodness of fit of the analytical model is in the Chap. 2 and many subsequent Chaps. With Cox regression AIC is not computed by SPSS statistical software. But it can be easily computed using the omnibus tests of coefficients as shown underneath for the data from our data example. Using the commands from the above Sect. 9.3 the computer will provide in the output sheets the underneath tables. The treatment modality is an insignificant predictor of survival at p = 0,147. Also Kaplan Meier curves were provided.

Omnibus Tests of Model Coefficients

-2 Log Likelihood
50,681

Omnibus Tests of Model Coefficients[a]

-2 Log Likelihood	Overall (score)			Change From Previous Step			Change From Previous Block		
	Chi-square	df	Sig.	Chi-square	df	Sig.	Chi-square	df	Sig.
48,506	2,205	1	,138	2,174	1	,140	2,174	1	,140

a. Beginning Block Number 1. Method = Enter

Variables in the Equation

	B	SE	Wald	df	Sig.	Exp(B)
group	-,855	,590	2,099	1	,147	,425

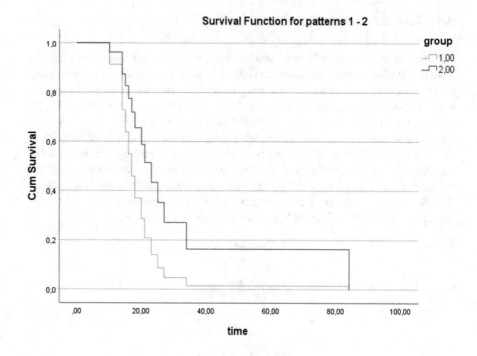

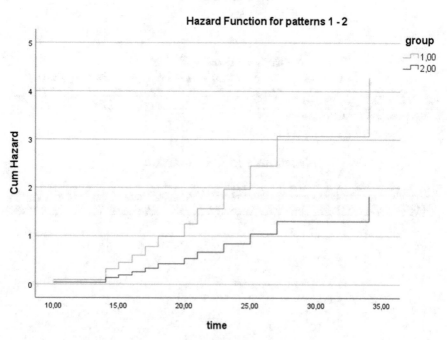

9.5   Accelerated Failure Time (AFT) Model with the Weibull Distribution

The output sheets provide the results from the Weibull AFT analysis.

Model Summary

Data Format	Nonrecurrent
Survival Time	time
Model	Accelerated failure time (AFT)
Model Distribution	Weibull
Feature Selection	None
Status	death
ADMM	Fast
Estimation Method	Automatically determined by the procedure

Model Fit Statistics

Log Likelihood	-11,293
-2 Log Likelihood	22,587
Akaike's Information Criterion (AIC)	28,587
Hurvich and Tsai's Criterion (AICC)	30,768
Schwarz's Bayesian Criterion (BIC)	30,711

AFT Model Regression Parameters

Parameter	Coefficient	Std. Error	Chi-Squared[a]	Sig.	95% Confidence Interval Lower	95% Confidence Interval Upper	Exp. Coefficient	Exp. 95% Confidence Interval Lower	Exp. 95% Confidence Interval Upper
Intercept	2,265	,401	31,882	<,001	1,479	3,051	9,628	4,387	21,132
group	,715	,271	6,975	,008	,184	1,246	2,045	1,203	3,477
(Scale)[b]	,488	,094	.	.	,335	,712	.	.	.

a. Degrees of freedom = 1

b. Chi-squared statistic, p-value, and the exponential statistics are not estimated for the scale parameter.

9.6   Accelerated Failure Time (AFT) Model with the Exponential Distribution

The output sheets provide the results of the exponential AFT analysis.

Model Summary

Data Format	Nonrecurrent
Survival Time	time
Model	Accelerated failure time (AFT)
Model Distribution	Exponential
Feature Selection	None
Status	death
ADMM	Fast
Estimation Method	Automatically determined by the procedure

Model Fit Statistics

Log Likelihood	-16,105
-2 Log Likelihood	32,210
Akaike's Information Criterion (AIC)	36,210
Hurvich and Tsai's Criterion (AICC)	37,210
Schwarz's Bayesian Criterion (BIC)	37,626

AFT Model Regression Parameters

Parameter	Coefficient	Std. Error	Chi-Squared[a]	Sig.	95% Confidence Interval		Exp. Coefficient	Exp. 95% Confidence Interval	
					Lower	Upper		Lower	Upper
Intercept	2,457	,816	9,055	,003	,857	4,057	11,670	2,355	57,818
group	,507	,540	,881	,348	-,552	1,565	1,660	,576	4,785
(Scale)[b]	1,000	.	.	.	.	.	.	.	.

a. Degrees of freedom = 1

b. Scale parameter is fixed at 1 for exponential distribution. Its related statistics are not estimated.

9.7   Accelerated Failure Time (AFT) Model with the Log Normal Distribution

The output sheets provide the results from the log normal AFT analysis.

Model Summary

Data Format	Nonrecurrent
Survival Time	time
Model	Accelerated failure time (AFT)
Model Distribution	Log-normal
Feature Selection	None
Status	death
ADMM	Fast
Estimation Method	Automatically determined by the procedure

Model Fit Statistics

Log Likelihood	-8,477
-2 Log Likelihood	16,954
Akaike's Information Criterion (AIC)	22,954
Hurvich and Tsai's Criterion (AICC)	25,136
Schwarz's Bayesian Criterion (BIC)	25,079

AFT Model Regression Parameters

Parameter	Coefficient	Std. Error	Chi-Squared[a]	Sig.	95% Confidence Interval Lower	95% Confidence Interval Upper	Exp. Coefficient	Exp. 95% Confidence Interval Lower	Exp. 95% Confidence Interval Upper
Intercept	2,415	,351	47,266	<,001	1,727	3,104	11,192	5,622	22,282
group	,435	,234	3,471	,062	-,023	,893	1,546	,978	2,443
(Scale)[b]	,436	,081	.	.	,302	,629	.	.	.

a. Degrees of freedom = 1
b. Chi-squared statistic, p-value, and the exponential statistics are not estimated for the scale parameter.

9.8   Accelerated Failure Time (AFT) Model with Log Logistic Distribution

The output sheets provide the log logistic AFT analysis.

Model Summary

Data Format	Nonrecurrent
Survival Time	time
Model	Accelerated failure time (AFT)
Model Distribution	Log-logistic
Feature Selection	None
Status	death
ADMM	Fast
Estimation Method	Automatically determined by the procedure

Model Fit Statistics

Log Likelihood	-7,667
-2 Log Likelihood	15,333
Akaike's Information Criterion (AIC)	21,333
Hurvich and Tsai's Criterion (AICC)	23,515
Schwarz's Bayesian Criterion (BIC)	23,458

AFT Model Regression Parameters

Parameter	Coefficient	Std. Error	Chi-Squared[a]	Sig.	95% Confidence Interval Lower	95% Confidence Interval Upper	Exp. Coefficient	Exp. 95% Confidence Interval Lower	Exp. 95% Confidence Interval Upper
Intercept	2,474	,294	70,810	<,001	1,898	3,050	11,866	6,669	21,113
group	,353	,198	3,166	,075	-,036	,742	1,423	,965	2,100
(Scale)[b]	,219	,051	.	.	,139	,346	.	.	.

a. Degrees of freedom = 1

b. Chi-squared statistic, p-value, and the exponential statistics are not estimated for the scale parameter.

9.9 Conclusion

	P-value of difference between treatments		Akaike Information Criterion
Cox	p = 0.138	NS (not significant)	48,508
Weibull	p = 0.008	S (significant)	28,587
Exponential	p = 0.348	NS	36,210
Log normal	p = 0.062	(S) (trend to S)	22,954
Log logistic	p = 0,075	(S)	21,333

Only the Weibull analysis provided a very significant result. The Cox regression was statistically insignificant.

References

Five textbooks complementary to the current production and written by the same authors are
(1) Statistics applied to clinical studies 5th edition, 2012,
(2) Machine learning in medicine a complete overview, 2020,
(3) Regression Analysis in Medical Research, 2nd Edition, 2021,
(4) Quantile regression in Clinical Research, 2021,
(5) Kernel Ridge Regression in Clinical research, 2022,
all of them edited by Springer Heidelberg Germany.

Chapter 10
The Effect on Survival from Stages 1 and 2 Histiocytic Lymphoma

Abstract In 81 patients with histiocytic lymphoma the disease stage was a significant predictor of survival at a p-value of 0,013 in the Cox regression. With the Accelerated failure time model with exponential distribution the p-value fell to 0,005. The effect of stage on survival was estimated in patients with stage 1 and stage 2 histiocytic lymphoma.

10.1 Introduction

Disease stage may influence survival. However prospective controlled studies with stage as endpoint are rare. In this chapter the effect on survival of stage 1 versus stage 2 will be assessed. Survival can be measured in the form of either a hazard, which is the ratio of deaths and non deaths in a random sample, or as a risk which is the proportion of deaths in the same sample. In this chapter hazard and risk of the same data will be computed in an 81 patient parallel group study using respectively Cox regression and Accelerated failure time models.

10.2 Data Example

The effect of stage on survival was estimated in patients with stage 1 and stage 2 histiocytic lymphoma.

Supplementary Information The online version contains supplementary material available at https://doi.org/10.1007/978-3-031-31632-6_10.

Stage	time	event (days)
1	6	1
1	19	1
1	32	1
1	42	1
1	42	1
1	43	0
1	94	1
1	126	0
1	169	0
1	207	1
1	211	0
1	227	0
1	253	1
1	255	0
1	270	0
1	310	0
1	316	0
1	335	0
1	346	0
2	4	1
2	6	1
2	10	1
2	11	1
2	11	1
2	11	1
2	13	1
2	17	1
2	20	1
2	20	1
2	21	1
2	22	1
2	24	1
2	24	1
2	29	1
2	30	1
2	30	1
2	31	1
2	33	1
2	34	1
2	35	1
2	39	1

(continued)

Stage	time	event (days)
2	40	1
2	41	0
2	43	0
2	45	1
2	46	1
2	50	1
2	56	1
2	61	0
2	61	0
2	63	1
2	68	1
2	82	1
2	85	1
2	88	1
2	89	1
2	90	1
2	93	1
2	104	1
2	110	1
2	134	1
2	137	1
2	160	0
2	169	1
2	171	1
2	173	1
2	175	1
2	184	1
2	201	1
2	222	1
2	235	0
2	247	0
2	260	0
2	284	0
2	290	0
2	291	0
2	302	0
2	304	0
2	341	0
2	345	0

10.3   Data Analysis Using SPSS Statistical Software
Version 29

The commands for Cox regression and for Accelerated failure time models are summarized underneath.

For convenience the data file entitled "Chapter 10,..." is in SpringerLink supplementary files. Start by opening the data file in your computer mounted with SPSS statistical software version 29.

For Cox regression click in the SPSS Menu:

Analyze....Survival....Cox Regression....time: enter time to event....status: enter event yes or no (1 or 0)....Define Event: enter 1....Covariates....click Categorical....Categorical Covariates: enter covariate....click Continue....click Plots....mark Survival....mark Hazard....click Continue....click OK.
For Accelerated failure times models click:

Analyze....Survival....Parametric Accelerated Failure Times (AFT) Models.... mark Survival....enter: "time" or "follow up mths" or "timetoevent"....status: enter event....click Define Event...default values are given: Failure/Event = 1, Right Censoring = 0, Left Censoring and Interval Censoring are not defined.... click Continue....Covariate(s) enter treatment, age, gender, etc....click Model: mark Distribution of Survival Time....mark Weibull....click Continue.... click OK.

In the output sheets several tables of the goodness of fit and p-values of statistical significance of various covariates are included.

10.4   Cox Regression

With Cox regression hazards and hazard ratios are computed (see also the Chap. 2). Also the Akaike Information Criterion (AIC) is computed. It is an important estimator the goodness of fit of a statistical analysis model. The smaller the AIC value the better the goodness of fit of the data. More information of the AICs (Akaike Information Criteria) as measure for goodness of fit of the analytical model is in the Chap. 2 and many subsequent Chaps. With Cox regression AIC is not computed by SPSS statistical software. But it can be easily computed using the omnibus tests of coefficients as shown underneath for the data from our data example. Using the commands from the above Sect. 10.3 the computer will provide in the output sheets the underneath tables. The disease stage is a significant predictor of survival at p = 0,013.

Omnibus Tests of Model Coefficients

-2 Log
Likelihood

415,110

Omnibus Tests of Model Coefficients[a]

-2 Log Likelihood	Overall (score)			Change From Previous Step			Change From Previous Block		
	Chi-square	df	Sig.	Chi-square	df	Sig.	Chi-square	df	Sig.
407,475	6,683	1	,010	7,634	1	,006	7,634	1	,006

a. Beginning Block Number 1. Method = Enter

Variables in the Equation

	B	SE	Wald	df	Sig.	Exp(B)
histiocytlymphoma	,961	,386	6,210	1	,013	2,614

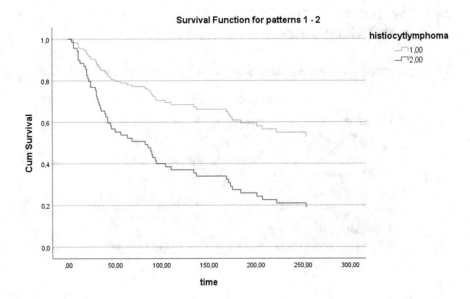

Survival Function for patterns 1 - 2

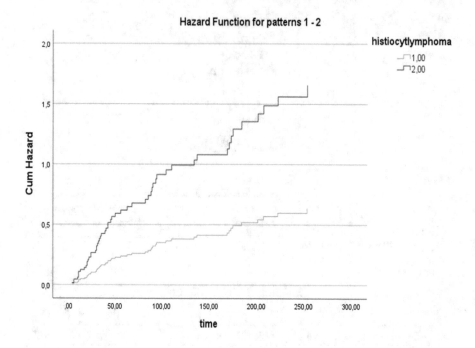

10.5 Accelerated Failure Time (AFT) with Weibull Distribution

The output sheets provide the results from the Weibull's AFT analysis.

Model Summary

Data Format	Nonrecurrent
Survival Time	time
Model	Accelerated failure time (AFT)
Model Distribution	Weibull
Feature Selection	None
Status	event
ADMM	Fast
Estimation Method	Automatically determined by the procedure

Model Fit Statistics

Log Likelihood	-122,153
-2 Log Likelihood	244,306
Akaike's Information Criterion (AIC)	250,306
Hurvich and Tsai's Criterion (AICC)	250,621
Schwarz's Bayesian Criterion (BIC)	257,452

AFT Model Regression Parameters

Parameter	Coefficient	Std. Error	Chi-Squared[a]	Sig.	95% Confidence Interval		Exp. Coefficient	Exp. 95% Confidence Interval	
					Lower	Upper		Lower	Upper
Intercept	7,386	,892	68,625	<,001	5,639	9,134	1613,659	281,099	9263,253
stage	-1,232	,472	6,811	,009	-2,158	-,307	,292	,116	,736
(Scale)[b]	1,208	,136	.	.	,969	1,507	.	.	.

a. Degrees of freedom = 1

b. Chi-squared statistic, p-value, and the exponential statistics are not estimated for the scale parameter.

10.6 Accelerated Failure Time (AFT) with Exponential Distribution

The output sheets provide the results from the exponential AFT analysis.

Model Summary

Data Format	Nonrecurrent
Survival Time	time
Model	Accelerated failure time (AFT)
Model Distribution	Exponential
Feature Selection	None
Status	event
ADMM	Fast
Estimation Method	Automatically determined by the procedure

Model Fit Statistics

Log Likelihood	-123,689
-2 Log Likelihood	247,378
Akaike's Information Criterion (AIC)	251,378
Hurvich and Tsai's Criterion (AICC)	251,534
Schwarz's Bayesian Criterion (BIC)	256,142

AFT Model Regression Parameters

Parameter	Coefficient	Std. Error	Chi-Squared[a]	Sig.	95% Confidence Interval		Exp. Coefficient	Exp. 95% Confidence Interval	
					Lower	Upper		Lower	Upper
Intercept	7,109	,722	96,852	<,001	5,693	8,524	1222,319	296,724	5035,191
stage	-1,085	,383	8,028	,005	-1,836	-,335	,338	,159	,716
(Scale)[b]	1,000	.	.	.	.	.	.	.	.

a. Degrees of freedom = 1

b. Scale parameter is fixed at 1 for exponential distribution. Its related statistics are not estimated.

10.7 Accelerated Failure Time (AFT) with Log Normal Distribution

The output sheets provide the results from the log normal AFT analysis.

Model Summary

Data Format	Nonrecurrent
Survival Time	time
Model	Accelerated failure time (AFT)
Model Distribution	Log-normal
Feature Selection	None
Status	event
ADMM	Fast
Estimation Method	Automatically determined by the procedure

Model Fit Statistics

Log Likelihood	-118,768
-2 Log Likelihood	237,536
Akaike's Information Criterion (AIC)	243,536
Hurvich and Tsai's Criterion (AICC)	243,852
Schwarz's Bayesian Criterion (BIC)	250,682

AFT Model Regression Parameters

Parameter	Coefficient	Std. Error	Chi-Squared[a]	Sig.	95% Confidence Interval		Exp. Coefficient	Exp. 95% Confidence Interval	
					Lower	Upper		Lower	Upper
Intercept	6,544	,811	65,072	<,001	4,954	8,133	694,769	141,697	3406,602
stage	-1,087	,438	6,165	,013	-1,945	-,229	,337	,143	,795
(Scale)[b]	1,484	,152	.	.	1,214	1,814	.	.	.

a. Degrees of freedom = 1

b. Chi-squared statistic, p-value, and the exponential statistics are not estimated for the scale parameter.

10.8   Accelerated Failure Time (AFT) with Log Logistic Distribution

The output sheets provide the results from the log logistic AFT aanalysis

Model Summary

Data Format	Nonrecurrent
Survival Time	time
Model	Accelerated failure time (AFT)
Model Distribution	Log-logistic
Feature Selection	None
Status	event
ADMM	Fast
Estimation Method	Automatically determined by the procedure

Model Fit Statistics

Log Likelihood	-119,521
-2 Log Likelihood	239,042
Akaike's Information Criterion (AIC)	245,042
Hurvich and Tsai's Criterion (AICC)	245,358
Schwarz's Bayesian Criterion (BIC)	252,188

AFT Model Regression Parameters

Parameter	Coefficient	Std. Error	Chi-Squared[a]	Sig.	95% Confidence Interval		Exp. Coefficient	Exp. 95% Confidence Interval	
					Lower	Upper		Lower	Upper
Intercept	6,806	,851	63,900	<,001	5,137	8,475	903,138	170,232	4791,436
stage	-1,239	,458	7,327	,007	-2,136	-,342	,290	,118	,710
(Scale)[b]	,878	,099	.	.	,703	1,095	.	.	.

a. Degrees of freedom = 1

b. Chi-squared statistic, p-value, and the exponential statistics are not estimated for the scale parameter.

10.9   Conclusion

	p-value of difference between stages	Akaike Information Criterion
Cox	p = 0,013,	407,477
Weibull	p = 0,009,	250,306
Exponential	p = 0,005,	251,378
Log normal	p = 0,013,	243,852
Log logistic	p = 0,007	245,042

The best p-values were by the AFT Exponential, Log logistic and Weibull distributions. The poorest p-value by the Cox and the AFT Log normal distribution. The AIC values were correspondingly better fit with the AFT models than they were with the Cox regression.

References

Five textbooks complementary to the current production and written by the same authors are
(1) Statistics applied to clinical studies 5th edition, 2012,
(2) Machine learning in medicine a complete overview, 2020,
(3) Regression Analysis in Medical Research, 2nd Edition, 2021,
(4) Quantile regression in Clinical Research, 2021,
(5) Kernel Ridge Regression in Clinical research, 2022
all of them edited by Springer Heidelberg Germany.

Chapter 11
Survival of 64 Lymphoma Patients with or Without B Symptoms

Abstract In 64 lymphoma patients the presence of B symptoms was a significant predictor of survival with a p-value of 0,007 in the Cox regression. In the Accelerated failure time models with both the exponential and the log logistics distributions the p-values fell to 0,001.

11.1 Introduction

The presence of B symptoms may be a predictor of poor survival. Documented proof in studies with B symptoms as endpoint is rare. In this chapter the effect on survival is assessed against that of the presence of only A symptoms. Survival can be measured in the form of either a hazard, which is the ratio of deaths and non-deaths in a random sample, or as a risk which is the proportion of deaths in the same sample. In this chapter hazard and risk of the same data will be computed in a 64 patient parallel group study using respectively Cox regression and Accelerated failure time models.

11.2 Data Example

The effect on survival of the presence of B symptoms or not in 64 lymphoma patients was analyzed.

Supplementary Information The online version contains supplementary material available at https://doi.org/10.1007/978-3-031-31632-6_11.

97

T. J. Cleophas, A. H. Zwinderman, *Modern Survival Analysis in Clinical Research*, https://doi.org/10.1007/978-3-031-31632-6_11

Months	Death	Symptoms (1 = A symptoms, 2 = B symptoms)
3,20	,00	1,00
4,40	,00	1,00
6,20	1,00	1,00
9,00	1,00	1,00
9,90	1,00	1,00
14,40	1,00	1,00
15,80	1,00	1,00
18,50	1,00	1,00
27,60	,00	1,00
28,50	1,00	1,00
30,10	,00	1,00
31,50	,00	1,00
32,20	,00	1,00
41,00	1,00	1,00
41,80	,00	1,00
44,50	,00	1,00
47,80	,00	1,00
50,60	,00	1,00
54,30	,00	1,00
55,00	1,00	1,00
60,00	,00	1,00
60,40	,00	1,00
63,60	,00	1,00
63,70	,00	1,00
63,80	,00	1,00
66,10	,00	1,00
68,00	,00	1,00
68,70	,00	1,00
68,80	,00	1,00
70,90	,00	1,00
71,50	,00	1,00
75,30	,00	1,00
2,50	1,00	2,00
4,10	1,00	2,00
4,60	1,00	2,00
6,40	1,00	2,00
6,70	1,00	2,00
7,40	1,00	2,00
7,60	1,00	2,00
7,70	1,00	2,00
7,80	1,00	2,00
8,80	1,00	2,00
13,30	1,00	2,00

(continued)

Months	Death	Symptoms (1 = A symptoms, 2 = B symptoms)
13,40	1,00	2,00
18,30	1,00	2,00
19,70	1,00	2,00
19,70	1,00	2,00
21,90	1,00	2,00
24,70	1,00	2,00
27,50	1,00	2,00
29,70	1,00	2,00
30,10	,00	2,00
32,90	1,00	2,00
33,50	,00	2,00
35,40	,00	2,00
37,70	,00	2,00
40,90	,00	2,00
42,60	,00	2,00
45,40	,00	2,00
48,50	,00	2,00
48,90	,00	2,00
60,40	,00	2,00
64,40	,00	2,00
66,40	,00	2,00

11.3   Data Analysis in SPSS Statistical Software Version 29

The commands for Cox regression and for Accelerated failure time models are summarized underneath.

For convenience the data file entitled "Chapter 11,…" is in SpringerLink supplementary files. Start by opening the data file in your computer mounted with SPSS statistical software version 29.

For Cox regression click in the SPSS Menu:

Analyze….Survival….Cox Regression….time: enter time to event….status: enter event yes or no (1 or 0)….Define Event: enter 1….Covariates….click Categorical….Categorical Covariates: enter covariate….click Continue….click Plots….mark Survival….mark Hazard….click Continue….click OK.

For Accelerated failure times models click:

Analyze….Survival….Parametric Accelerated Failure Times (AFT) Models…. mark Survival….enter: "time" or "follow up mths" or "timetoevent"….status: enter event….click Define Event…default values are given: Failure/Event = 1, Right Censoring = 0, Left Censoring and Interval Censoring are not defined…. click Continue….Covariate(s) enter treatment, age, gender, etc….click Model: mark Distribution of Survival Time….mark Weibull….click Continue…. click OK.

In the output sheets several tables of the goodness of fit and p-values of statistical significance of various covariates are included.

11.4   Cox Regression

With Cox regression hazards and hazard ratios are computed (see also the Chap. 2). Also the Akaike Information Criterion (AIC) is computed. It is an important estimator the goodness of fit of a statistical analysis model. The smaller the AIC value the better the goodness of fit of the data. More information of the AICs (Akaike Information Criteria) as measure for goodness of fit of the analytical model is in the Chap. 2 and many subsequent Chaps. With Cox regression AIC is not computed by SPSS statistical software. But it can be easily computed using the omnibus tests of coefficients as shown underneath for the data from our data example. Using the commands from the above Sect. 11.3 the computer will provide in the output sheets the underneath tables. The presence of B symptoms is a significant predictor of survival at p = 0,007.

Omnibus Tests of Model Coefficients

-2 Log Likelihood
221,257

Omnibus Tests of Model Coefficients[a]

-2 Log Likelihood	Overall (score)			Change From Previous Step			Change From Previous Block		
	Chi-square	df	Sig.	Chi-square	df	Sig.	Chi-square	df	Sig.
213,171	8,091	1	,004	8,087	1	,004	8,087	1	,004

a. Beginning Block Number 1. Method = Enter

Variables in the Equation

	B	SE	Wald	df	Sig.	Exp(B)
group	1,101	,406	7,362	1	,007	3,009

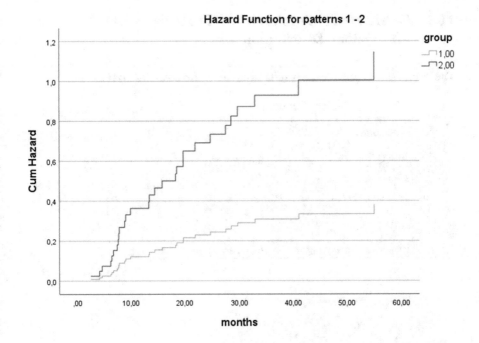

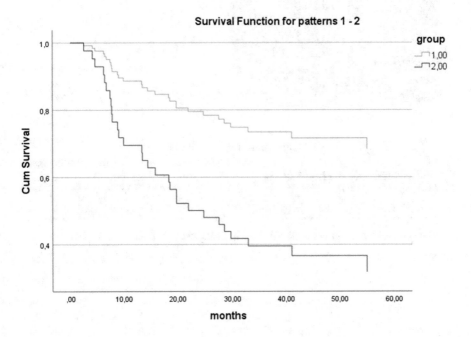

11.5   Accelerated Failure Time (AFT) Model with Weibull Distribution

The output sheets provide the results from the Weibull AFT analysis.

Model Summary

Data Format	Nonrecurrent
Survival Time	months
Model	Accelerated failure time (AFT)
Model Distribution	Weibull
Feature Selection	None
Status	event
ADMM	Fast
Estimation Method	Automatically determined by the procedure

Model Fit Statistics

Log Likelihood	-74,664
-2 Log Likelihood	149,328
Akaike's Information Criterion (AIC)	155,328
Hurvich and Tsai's Criterion (AICC)	155,728
Schwarz's Bayesian Criterion (BIC)	161,805

AFT Model Regression Parameters

Parameter	Coefficient	Std. Error	Chi-Squared[a]	Sig.	95% Confidence Interval		Exp. Coefficient	Exp. 95% Confidence Interval	
					Lower	Upper		Lower	Upper
Intercept	6,446	,826	60,880	<,001	4,827	8,066	630,428	124,849	3183,370
group	-1,347	,455	8,774	,003	-2,239	-,456	,260	,107	,634
(Scale)[b]	1,069	,173	.	.	,778	1,469	.	.	.

a. Degrees of freedom = 1

b. Chi-squared statistic, p-value, and the exponential statistics are not estimated for the scale parameter.

11.6   Accelerated Failure Time (AFT) Model with Exponential Distribution

The output sheets provide the results from the exponential AFT analysis.

Model Summary

Data Format	Nonrecurrent
Survival Time	months
Model	Accelerated failure time (AFT)
Model Distribution	Exponential
Feature Selection	None
Status	event
ADMM	Fast
Estimation Method	Automatically determined by the procedure

Model Fit Statistics

Log Likelihood	-74,751
-2 Log Likelihood	149,503
Akaike's Information Criterion (AIC)	153,503
Hurvich and Tsai's Criterion (AICC)	153,699
Schwarz's Bayesian Criterion (BIC)	157,820

AFT Model Regression Parameters

Parameter	Coefficient	Std. Error	Chi-Squared[a]	Sig.	95% Confidence Interval		Exp. Coefficient	Exp. 95% Confidence Interval	
					Lower	Upper		Lower	Upper
Intercept	6,310	,703	80,529	<,001	4,932	7,688	550,074	138,640	2182,503
group	-1,287	,401	10,279	,001	-2,074	-,500	,276	,126	,606
(Scale)[b]	1,000	.	.	.	.	.	.	.	.

a. Degrees of freedom = 1

b. Scale parameter is fixed at 1 for exponential distribution. Its related statistics are not estimated.

11.7   Accelerated Failure Time (AFT) Model with Log Normal Distribution

The output sheets provide the results from the log normal AFT analysis.

Model Summary

Data Format	Nonrecurrent
Survival Time	months
Model	Accelerated failure time (AFT)
Model Distribution	Log-normal
Feature Selection	None
Status	event
ADMM	Fast
Estimation Method	Automatically determined by the procedure

Model Fit Statistics

Log Likelihood	-71,923
-2 Log Likelihood	143,846
Akaike's Information Criterion (AIC)	149,846
Hurvich and Tsai's Criterion (AICC)	150,246
Schwarz's Bayesian Criterion (BIC)	156,323

AFT Model Regression Parameters

Parameter	Coefficient	Std. Error	Chi-Squared[a]	Sig.	95% Confidence Interval		Exp. Coefficient	Exp. 95% Confidence Interval	
					Lower	Upper		Lower	Upper
Intercept	5,945	,733	65,707	<,001	4,508	7,383	381,912	90,712	1607,909
group	-1,322	,423	9,773	,002	-2,150	-,493	,267	,116	,611
(Scale)[b]	1,409	,207	.	.	1,057	1,879	.		

a. Degrees of freedom = 1

b. Chi-squared statistic, p-value, and the exponential statistics are not estimated for the scale parameter.

11.8   Accelerated Failure Time (AFT) Model with Log Logistic Distribution

The output sheets provide the results from the log logistic AFT analysis.

Model Summary

Data Format	Nonrecurrent
Survival Time	months
Model	Accelerated failure time (AFT)
Model Distribution	Log-logistic
Feature Selection	None
Status	event
ADMM	Fast
Estimation Method	Automatically determined by the procedure

Model Fit Statistics

Log Likelihood	-72,953
-2 Log Likelihood	145,905
Akaike's Information Criterion (AIC)	151,905
Hurvich and Tsai's Criterion (AICC)	152,305
Schwarz's Bayesian Criterion (BIC)	158,382

AFT Model Regression Parameters

Parameter	Coefficient	Std. Error	Chi-Squared[a]	Sig.	95% Confidence Interval		Exp. Coefficient	Exp. 95% Confidence Interval	
					Lower	Upper		Lower	Upper
Intercept	6,053	,754	64,407	<,001	4,574	7,531	425,202	96,970	1864,451
group	-1,405	,436	10,399	,001	-2,260	-,551	,245	,104	,576
(Scale)[b]	,841	,133	.	.	,617	1,146	.	.	.

a. Degrees of freedom = 1

b. Chi-squared statistic, p-value, and the exponential statistics are not estimated for the scale parameter.

11.9   Conclusion

	P-value of difference B symptoms or not	Akaike Information Criterion
Cox	p = 0,007,	213,173
AFT weibull	p = 0,003,	155,328
AFT exponential	p = 0,001,	151,503
AFT log normal	p = 0,002,	149,846
AFT log logistic	p = 0,001	151,905

All of the AFT p-values and AFT Akaike information criteria are better than those of the Cox regression.

References

Five textbooks complementary to the current production and written by the same authors are
(1) Statistics applied to clinical studies 5th edition, 2012,
(2) Machine learning in medicine a complete overview, 2020,
(3) Regression Analysis in Medical Research, 2nd Edition, 2021,
(4) Quantile regression in Clinical Research, 2021,
(5) Kernel Ridge Regression in Clinical research, 2022,
all of them edited by Springer Heidelberg Germany.

Chapter 12
Effect on Time-to-Event of Group Membership

Abstract In 18 patients the group membership was an insignificant predictor of event with a p-value of 0,058 in the Cox regression. With the Accelerated failure time model with Weibull distribution the p-value fell to 0,008.

12.1 Introduction

There are often clinical arguments to support that group membership may influence survival. However documented proof is often missing. In this chapter the effect on survival of group membership is assessed. Survival can be measured in the form of either a hazard, which is the ratio of deaths and non-deaths in a random sample, or as a risk which is the proportion of deaths in the same sample. In this chapter hazard and risk of the same data will be computed in an 18 patient parallel group study using respectively Cox regression and Accelerated failure time models.

12.2 Data Example

A data example from the site of "graphpad.com_stat_howto-survival" was used. The effect on time-to-event of being in a group was measured in 18 patients.

Time (days)	event	group
34,00	1,00	1,00
66,00	1,00	1,00
64,00	,00	1,00
89,00	1,00	1,00

(continued)

Supplementary Information The online version contains supplementary material available at https://doi.org/10.1007/978-3-031-31632-6_12.

T. J. Cleophas, A. H. Zwinderman, *Modern Survival Analysis in Clinical Research*, https://doi.org/10.1007/978-3-031-31632-6_12

Time (days)	event	group
98,00	1,00	1,00
111,00	1,00	1,00
123,00	1,00	1,00
145,00	,00	1,00
88,00	1,00	2,00
143,00	1,00	2,00
76,00	1,00	2,00
111,00	,00	2,00
95,00	,00	2,00
134,00	1,00	2,00
167,00	1,00	2,00
198,00	1,00	2,00
211,00	1,00	2,00
234,00	1,00	2,00

12.3   Data Analysis Using SPSS Statistical Software Version 29

The commands for Cox regression and for Accelerated failure time models are summarized underneath.

For convenience the data file entitled "Chapter 12,......" is in SpringerLink supplementary files. Start by opening the data file in your computer mounted with SPSS statistical software version 29.

For Cox regression click in the SPSS Menu:

Analyze....Survival....Cox Regression....time: enter time to event....status: enter event yes or no (1 or 0)....Define Event: enter 1....Covariates....click Categorical....Categorical Covariates: enter covariate....click Continue....click Plots....mark Survival....mark Hazard....click Continue....click OK.

For Accelerated failure times models click:

Analyze....Survival....Parametric Accelerated Failure Times (AFT) Models.... mark Survival....enter: "time" or "follow up mths" or "timetoevent"....status: enter event....click Define Event...default values are given: Failure/Event = 1, Right Censoring = 0, Left Censoring and Interval Censoring are not defined.... click Continue....Covariate(s) enter treatment, age, gender, etc....click Model: mark Distribution of Survival Time....mark Weibull....click Continue.... click OK.

In the output sheets several tables of the goodness of fit and p-values of statistical significance of various covariates are included.

12.4 Cox Regression

With Cox regression hazards and hazard ratios are computed (see also the Chap. 2).
Also the Akaike Information Criterion (AIC) is computed. It is an important estimator the goodness of fit of a statistical analysis model. The smaller the AIC value the
better the goodness of fit of the data. More information of the AICs (Akaike
Information Criteria) as measure for goodness of fit of the analytical model is in the
Chap. 2 and many subsequent Chaps. With Cox regression AIC is not computed by
SPSS statistical software. But it can be easily computed using the omnibus tests of
coefficients as shown underneath for the data from our data example. Using the
commands from the above Sect. 12.3 the computer will provide in the output sheets
the underneath tables. The group membership is an insignificant predictor of survival at p = 0,058.

Omnibus Tests of Model Coefficients

-2 Log Likelihood
54,541

Omnibus Tests of Model Coefficients[a]

-2 Log Likelihood	Overall (score)			Change From Previous Step			Change From Previous Block		
	Chi-square	df	Sig.	Chi-square	df	Sig.	Chi-square	df	Sig.
50,852	4,033	1	,045	3,689	1	,055	3,689	1	,055

a. Beginning Block Number 1. Method = Enter

Variables in the Equation

	B	SE	Wald	df	Sig.	Exp(B)
group	-1,260	,664	3,600	1	,058	,284

12.5   Accelerated Failure Time (AFT) Model with Weibull Distribution

The output sheets provide the results from the Weibull's AFT analysis.

Model Summary

Data Format	Nonrecurrent
Survival Time	time
Model	Accelerated failure time (AFT)
Model Distribution	Weibull
Feature Selection	None
Status	event
ADMM	Fast
Estimation Method	Automatically determined by the procedure

Model Fit Statistics

Log Likelihood	-9,021
-2 Log Likelihood	18,041
Akaike's Information Criterion (AIC)	24,041
Hurvich and Tsai's Criterion (AICC)	25,756
Schwarz's Bayesian Criterion (BIC)	26,713

AFT Model Regression Parameters

Parameter	Coefficient	Std. Error	Chi-Squared[a]	Sig.	95% Confidence Interval Lower	95% Confidence Interval Upper	Exp. Coefficient	Exp. 95% Confidence Interval Lower	Exp. 95% Confidence Interval Upper
Intercept	4,276	,278	236,066	<,001	3,730	4,821	71,936	41,693	124,116
group	,448	,169	7,036	,008	,117	,780	1,566	1,124	2,181
(Scale)[b]	,313	,066			,206	,474			

a. Degrees of freedom = 1

b. Chi-squared statistic, p-value, and the exponential statistics are not estimated for the scale parameter.

12.6   Accelerated Failure Time (AFT) with Exponential Distribution

The output sheets provide the results from the exponential AFT analysis.

Model Summary

Data Format	Nonrecurrent
Survival Time	time
Model	Accelerated failure time (AFT)
Model Distribution	Exponential
Feature Selection	None
Status	event
ADMM	Fast
Estimation Method	Automatically determined by the procedure

Model Fit Statistics

Log Likelihood	-18,252
-2 Log Likelihood	36,503
Akaike's Information Criterion (AIC)	40,503
Hurvich and Tsai's Criterion (AICC)	41,303
Schwarz's Bayesian Criterion (BIC)	42,284

AFT Model Regression Parameters

Parameter	Coefficient	Std. Error	Chi-Squared[a]	Sig.	95% Confidence Interval Lower	95% Confidence Interval Upper	Exp. Coefficient	Exp. 95% Confidence Interval Lower	Exp. 95% Confidence Interval Upper
Intercept	4,398	,890	24,431	<,001	2,654	6,142	81,275	14,210	464,851
group	,403	,540	,558	,455	-,655	1,462	1,497	,519	4,314
(Scale)[b]	1,000	.	.	.	.	.	.	.	.

a. Degrees of freedom = 1

b. Scale parameter is fixed at 1 for exponential distribution. Its related statistics are not estimated.

12.7   Accelerated Failure Time (AFT) with Log Normal Distribution

The output sheets provide the results from the log normal AFT analysis.

Model Summary

Data Format	Nonrecurrent
Survival Time	time
Model	Accelerated failure time (AFT)
Model Distribution	Log-normal
Feature Selection	None
Status	event
ADMM	Fast
Estimation Method	Automatically determined by the procedure

Model Fit Statistics

Log Likelihood	-10,096
-2 Log Likelihood	20,191
Akaike's Information Criterion (AIC)	26,191
Hurvich and Tsai's Criterion (AICC)	27,905
Schwarz's Bayesian Criterion (BIC)	28,862

AFT Model Regression Parameters

Parameter	Coefficient	Std. Error	Chi-Squared[a]	Sig.	95% Confidence Interval Lower	95% Confidence Interval Upper	Exp. Coefficient	Exp. 95% Confidence Interval Lower	Exp. 95% Confidence Interval Upper
Intercept	4,024	,349	133,064	<,001	3,340	4,708	55,916	28,224	110,780
group	,498	,214	5,412	,020	,078	,918	1,646	1,082	2,504
(Scale)[b]	,426	,080	.	.	,295	,615	.	.	.

a. Degrees of freedom = 1

b. Chi-squared statistic, p-value, and the exponential statistics are not estimated for the scale parameter.

12.8   Accelerated Failure Time (AFT) with Log Logistic Distribution

The output sheets provide the results from the log logistic AFT analysis.

Model Summary

Data Format	Nonrecurrent
Survival Time	time
Model	Accelerated failure time (AFT)
Model Distribution	Log-logistic
Feature Selection	None
Status	event
ADMM	Fast
Estimation Method	Automatically determined by the procedure

Model Fit Statistics

Log Likelihood	-9,995
-2 Log Likelihood	19,990
Akaike's Information Criterion (AIC)	25,990
Hurvich and Tsai's Criterion (AICC)	27,704
Schwarz's Bayesian Criterion (BIC)	28,661

AFT Model Regression Parameters

Parameter	Coefficient	Std. Error	Chi-Squared[a]	Sig.	95% Confidence Interval Lower	95% Confidence Interval Upper	Exp. Coefficient	Exp. 95% Confidence Interval Lower	Exp. 95% Confidence Interval Upper
Intercept	4,091	,339	145,480	<,001	3,426	4,756	59,787	30,755	116,226
group	,477	,208	5,230	,022	,068	,885	1,611	1,071	2,424
(Scale)[b]	,239	,052	.	.	,156	,367			

a. Degrees of freedom = 1

b. Chi-squared statistic, p-value, and the exponential statistics are not estimated for the scale parameter.

12.9   Conclusion

	p-value of difference between 2 groups	Akaike Information Criterion
Cox	0,058	50,854
Weibull	0,008	24,041
Exponential	0,455	40,503
Log normal	0,020	26,191
Log logistic	0,022	25,990

The Weibull p-value was very significant at $p = 0,008$, the Cox regression p-value was insignificant at $p = 0,058$.

References

Five textbooks complementary to the current production and written by the same authors are
(1) Statistics applied to clinical studies 5th edition, 2012,
(2) Machine learning in medicine a complete overview, 2020,
(3) Regression Analysis in Medical Research, 2nd Edition, 2021,
(4) Quantile regression in Clinical Research, 2021,
(5) Kernel Ridge Regression in Clinical research, 2022,
all of them edited by Springer Heidelberg Germany.

Chapter 13
The Effect on Survival of Group Membership

Abstract In 12 patients the group membership was an insignificant predictor of event with a p-value of 0,109 in the Cox regression. With the Accelerated failure time model with a log normal distribution the p-value fell to 0,047, and became thus statistically significant at $p < 0.05$.

13.1 Introduction

There are often clinical arguments to support that group membership may influence survival. However documented proof is often missing. In this chapter the effect on survival of group membership is assessed. Survival can be measured in the form of either a hazard, which is the ratio of deaths and non-deaths in a random sample, or as a risk which is the proportion of deaths in the same sample. In this chapter hazard and risk of the same data will be computed in a 12 patient parallel group study using respectively Cox regression and Accelerated failure time models.

13.2 Data Example

A data example from the site "graphpad.com_stat_howto_survival" was used. The effect on time-to-event of being in a group was measured in 18 patients.

Data are from the Practicle Guide to Understanding Kaplan-Meier Curves in Otolaryngeal Head Neck Surgery, in Head Neck Surgery 2010: 143; 331.

Supplementary Information The online version contains supplementary material available at https://doi.org/10.1007/978-3-031-31632-6_13.

T. J. Cleophas, A. H. Zwinderman, *Modern Survival Analysis in Clinical Research*, https://doi.org/10.1007/978-3-031-31632-6_13

Time	Event	Group membership
1,00	1,00	1,00
2,00	1,00	1,00
3,00	1,00	1,00
4,00	1,00	1,00
4,50	1,00	1,00
5,00	,00	1,00
,50	1,00	2,00
,75	1,00	2,00
1,00	1,00	2,00
1,50	,00	2,00
2,00	1,00	2,00
3,50	1,00	2,00

13.3   Data Analysis Using SPSS Statistical Software Version 29

The commands for Cox regression and for Accelerated failure time models are summarized underneath.

For convenience the data file entitled "Chapter 13,......" is in SpringerLink supplementary files. Start by opening the data file in your computer mounted with SPSS statistical software version 29.

For Cox regression click in the SPSS Menu:

Analyze....Survival....Cox Regression....time: enter time to event....status: enter event yes or no (1 or 0)....Define Event: enter 1....Covariates....click Categorical....Categorical Covariates: enter covariate....click Continue....click Plots....mark Survival....mark Hazard....click Continue....click OK.

For Accelerated failure times models click:

Analyze....Survival....Parametric Accelerated Failure Times (AFT) Models.... mark Survival....enter: "time" or "follow up mths" or "timetoevent"....status: enter event....click Define Event...default values are given: Failure/Event = 1, Right Censoring = 0, Left Censoring and Interval Censoring are not defined.... click Continue....Covariate(s) enter treatment, age, gender, etc....click Model: mark Distribution of Survival Time....mark Weibull....click Continue.... click OK.

In the output sheets several tables of the goodness of fit and p-values of statistical significance of various covariates are included.

13.4   Cox Regression

With Cox regression hazards and hazard ratios are computed (see also the Chap. 2).
Also the Akaike Information Criterion (AIC) is computed. It is an important estimator the goodness of fit of a statistical analysis model. The smaller the AIC value the
better the goodness of fit of the data. More information of the AICs (Akaike
Information Criteria) as measure for goodness of fit of the analytical model is in the
Chap. 2 and many subsequent Chaps. With Cox regression AIC is not computed by
SPSS statistical software. But it can be easily calculated using the omnibus tests of
coefficients as shown underneath for the data from our data example. Using the
commands from the above Sect. 13.3 the computer will provide in the output sheets
the underneath tables. The group membership is an insignificant predictor of survival at p = 0,109.

Omnibus Tests of Model Coefficients

-2 Log Likelihood
36,335

Omnibus Tests of Model Coefficients[a]

-2 Log Likelihood	Overall (score)			Change From Previous Step			Change From Previous Block		
	Chi-square	df	Sig.	Chi-square	df	Sig.	Chi-square	df	Sig.
33,653	2,853	1	,091	2,682	1	,101	2,682	1	,101

a. Beginning Block Number 1. Method = Enter

Variables in the Equation

	B	SE	Wald	df	Sig.	Exp(B)
group	1,200	,748	2,575	1	,109	3,319

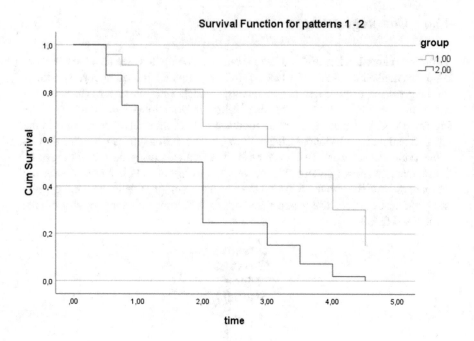

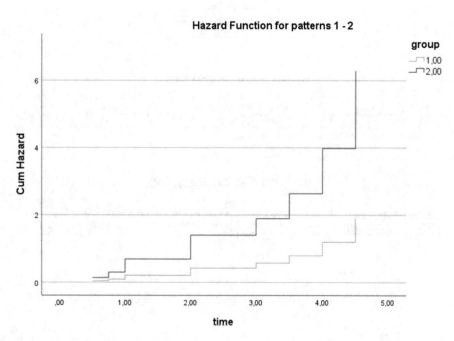

13.5   Accelerated Failure Time (AFT) Models with Weibull Distribution

The output sheets provide the results from the Weibull AFT analysis.

Model Summary

Data Format	Nonrecurrent
Survival Time	time
Model	Accelerated failure time (AFT)
Model Distribution	Weibull
Feature Selection	None
Status	event
ADMM	Fast
Estimation Method	Automatically determined by the procedure

Model Fit Statistics

Log Likelihood	-12,231
-2 Log Likelihood	24,461
Akaike's Information Criterion (AIC)	30,461
Hurvich and Tsai's Criterion (AICC)	33,461
Schwarz's Bayesian Criterion (BIC)	31,916

AFT Model Regression Parameters

Parameter	Coefficient	Std. Error	Chi-Squared[a]	Sig.	95% Confidence Interval		Exp. Coefficient	Exp. 95% Confidence Interval	
					Lower	Upper		Lower	Upper
Intercept	2,025	,562	12,969	<,001	,923	3,127	7,577	2,517	22,812
group	-,674	,357	3,557	,059	-1,374	,026	,510	,253	1,027
(Scale)[b]	,561	,143	.	.	,341	,924	.	.	.

a. Degrees of freedom = 1

b. Chi-squared statistic, p-value, and the exponential statistics are not estimated for the scale parameter.

13.6   Accelerated Failure Time (AFT) Models with Exponential Distribution

The output sheets provide the exponential AFT analysis.

Model Summary

Data Format	Nonrecurrent
Survival Time	time
Model	Accelerated failure time (AFT)
Model Distribution	Exponential
Feature Selection	None
Status	event
ADMM	Fast
Estimation Method	Automatically determined by the procedure

Model Fit Statistics

Log Likelihood	-14,234
-2 Log Likelihood	28,467
Akaike's Information Criterion (AIC)	32,467
Hurvich and Tsai's Criterion (AICC)	33,801
Schwarz's Bayesian Criterion (BIC)	33,437

AFT Model Regression Parameters

Parameter	Coefficient	Std. Error	Chi-Squared[a]	Sig.	95% Confidence Interval		Exp. Coefficient	Exp. 95% Confidence Interval	
					Lower	Upper		Lower	Upper
Intercept	2,107	1,000	4,438	,035	,147	4,067	8,221	1,158	58,360
group	-,746	,632	1,390	,238	-1,985	,494	,474	,137	1,639
(Scale)[b]	1,000	.	.	.	.	.	.	.	.

a. Degrees of freedom = 1

b. Scale parameter is fixed at 1 for exponential distribution. Its related statistics are not estimated.

13.7   Accelerated Failure Time (AFT) Model with Log Normal Distribution

The output sheets provide the results from the log normal AFT analysis.

Model Summary

Data Format	Nonrecurrent
Survival Time	time
Model	Accelerated failure time (AFT)
Model Distribution	Log-normal
Feature Selection	None
Status	event
ADMM	Fast
Estimation Method	Automatically determined by the procedure

Model Fit Statistics

Log Likelihood	-12,077
-2 Log Likelihood	24,154
Akaike's Information Criterion (AIC)	30,154
Hurvich and Tsai's Criterion (AICC)	33,154
Schwarz's Bayesian Criterion (BIC)	31,608

AFT Model Regression Parameters

Parameter	Coefficient	Std. Error	Chi-Squared[a]	Sig.	95% Confidence Interval		Exp. Coefficient	Exp. 95% Confidence Interval	
					Lower	Upper		Lower	Upper
Intercept	1,916	,636	9,079	,003	,670	3,163	6,795	1,954	23,632
group	-,801	,403	3,951	,047	-1,591	-,011	,449	,204	,989
(Scale)[b]	,681	,156	.	.	,435	1,067	.	.	.

a. Degrees of freedom = 1

b. Chi-squared statistic, p-value, and the exponential statistics are not estimated for the scale parameter.

13.8   Accelerated Failure Time (AFT) Model with Log Logistics Distribution

The output sheets provide the results from the log logistic AFT analysis.

Model Summary

Data Format	Nonrecurrent
Survival Time	time
Model	Accelerated failure time (AFT)
Model Distribution	Log-logistic
Feature Selection	None
Status	event
ADMM	Fast
Estimation Method	Automatically determined by the procedure

Model Fit Statistics

Log Likelihood	-12,436
-2 Log Likelihood	24,871
Akaike's Information Criterion (AIC)	30,871
Hurvich and Tsai's Criterion (AICC)	33,871
Schwarz's Bayesian Criterion (BIC)	32,326

AFT Model Regression Parameters

Parameter	Coefficient	Std. Error	Chi-Squared[a]	Sig.	95% Confidence Interval		Exp. Coefficient	Exp. 95% Confidence Interval	
					Lower	Upper		Lower	Upper
Intercept	1,987	,657	9,150	,002	,700	3,275	7,296	2,013	26,444
group	-,840	,427	3,864	,049	-1,678	-,002	,432	,187	,998
(Scale)[b]	,412	,106	.	.	,248	,684	.	.	.

a. Degrees of freedom = 1

b. Chi-squared statistic, p-value, and the exponential statistics are not estimated for the scale parameter.

13.9 Conclusion

	p-values between groups	Akaike Information Criterion (AIC)
Cox	0,109,	33,655
Weibull	0,059,	30,461
Exponential	0,238,	32,461
Log normal	0,047,	30,154
Log logistics	0,049	30,871

Three of four AFT (accelerated failure time) models provided p-values close to 0,05, while the Cox regression was insignificant at $p = 0,109$. Akaike values had corresponding magnitudes, the smaller the AIC the better the p-value. AFT models thus performed better than did Cox regression.

References

Five textbooks complementary to the current production and written by the same authors are
(1) Statistics applied to clinical studies 5th edition, 2012,
(2) Machine learning in medicine a complete overview, 2020,
(3) Regression Analysis in Medical Research, 2nd Edition, 2021,
(4) Quantile regression in Clinical Research, 2021,
(5) Kernel Ridge Regression in Clinical research, 2022,
all of them edited by Springer Heidelberg Germany.

Chapter 14
Deaths from Carcinoma After Exposure to Carcinogens in Rats

Abstract In 38 rats the exposure to carcinogens was an insignificant predictor of deaths from carcinoma with a p-value of 0,141 in the Cox regression. With the Accelerated failure time model with Weibull distribution the p-value fell to 0,050.

14.1 Introduction

There are often clinical arguments to support that exposure to carcinogens may influence survival. However documented proof is often missing. In this chapter the effect on survival of carcinogen exposure is assessed. Survival can be measured in the form of either a hazard, which is the ratio of deaths and non deaths in a random sample, or as a risk which is the proportion of deaths in the same sample. In this chapter hazard and risk of the same data will be computed in a 38 rat parallel group study using respectively Cox regression and Accelerated failure time models.

14.2 Data Example

Deaths from carcinoma after exposure to carcinogens are measured in two groups of rats. The dataset in this Chap. are from: Statsdirect.com/help/survival_analysis_kaplan-meier.htm.

Supplementary Information The online version contains supplementary material available at https://doi.org/10.1007/978-3-031-31632-6_14.

Time (hours)	event	group
143,00	1,00	1,00
165,00	1,00	1,00
188,00	1,00	1,00
188,00	1,00	1,00
190,00	1,00	1,00
192,00	1,00	1,00
206,00	1,00	1,00
208,00	1,00	1,00
212,00	1,00	1,00
220,00	1,00	1,00
227,00	1,00	1,00
230,00	1,00	1,00
235,00	1,00	1,00
246,00	1,00	1,00
265,00	1,00	1,00
303,00	1,00	1,00
216,00	,00	1,00
244,00	,00	1,00
142,00	1,00	2,00
157,00	1,00	2,00
163,00	1,00	2,00
198,00	1,00	2,00
205,00	1,00	2,00
232,00	1,00	2,00
233,00	1,00	2,00
233,00	1,00	2,00
233,00	1,00	2,00
233,00	1,00	2,00
239,00	1,00	2,00
240,00	1,00	2,00
261,00	1,00	2,00
280,00	1,00	2,00
295,00	1,00	2,00
295,00	1,00	2,00
323,00	1,00	2,00
204,00	,00	2,00
344,00	,00	2,00

14.3 Data Analysis Using SPSS Statistical Software Version 29

The commands for Cox regression and for Accelerated failure time models are summarized underneath.

For convenience the data file entitled "Chapter 14,......" is in SpringerLink supplementary files. Start by opening the data file in your computer mounted with SPSS statistical software version 29.

For Cox regression click in the SPSS Menu:

Analyze....Survival....Cox Regression....time: enter time to event....status: enter event yes or no (1 or 0)....Define Event: enter 1....Covariates....click Categorical....Categorical Covariates: enter covariate....click Continue....click Plots....mark Survival....mark Hazard....click Continue....click OK.

For Accelerated failure times models click:

Analyze....Survival....Parametric Accelerated Failure Times (AFT) Models....mark Survival....enter: "time" or "follow up mths" or "timetoevent"....status: enter event....click Define Event...default values are given: Failure/Event = 1, Right Censoring = 0, Left Censoring and Interval Censoring are not defined....click Continue....Covariate(s) enter treatment, age, gender, etc....click Model: mark Distribution of Survival Time....mark Weibull....click Continue....click OK.

In the output sheets several tables of the goodness of fit and p-values of statistical significance of various covariates are included.

14.4 Cox Regression

With Cox regression hazards and hazard ratios are computed (see also the Chap. 2). Also the Akaike Information Criterion (AIC) is computed. It is an important estimator the goodness of fit of a statistical analysis model. The smaller the AIC value the better the goodness of fit of the data. More information of the AICs (Akaike Information Criteria) as measure for goodness of fit of the analytical model is in the Chap. 2 and many subsequent Chaps. With Cox regression AIC is not computed by SPSS statistical software. But it can be easily calculated using the omnibus tests of coefficients as shown underneath for the data from our data example. Using the commands from the above Sect. 14.3 the computer will provide in the output sheets the underneath tables. The carcinogen exposure is an insignificant predictor of survival at p = 0,141.

Omnibus Tests of Model Coefficients

-2 Log Likelihood
182,552

Omnibus Tests of Model Coefficients[a]

-2 Log Likelihood	Overall (score)			Change From Previous Step			Change From Previous Block		
	Chi-square	df	Sig.	Chi-square	df	Sig.	Chi-square	df	Sig.
180,407	2,210	1	,137	2,145	1	,143	2,145	1	,143

a. Beginning Block Number 1. Method = Enter

Variables in the Equation

	B	SE	Wald	df	Sig.	Exp(B)
group	-,533	,362	2,165	1	,141	,587

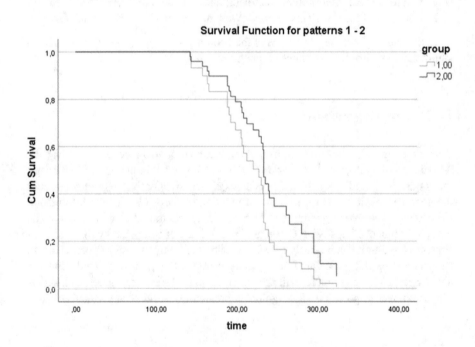

Survival Function for patterns 1 - 2

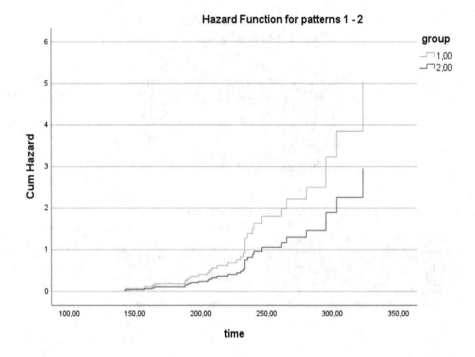

14.5   Accelerated Failure Time (AFT) Model with Weibull Distribution

The output sheets provide the results from the Weibull's AFT analysis.

Model Summary

Data Format	Nonrecurrent
Survival Time	time
Model	Accelerated failure time (AFT)
Model Distribution	Weibull
Feature Selection	None
Status	event
ADMM	Fast
Estimation Method	Automatically determined by the procedure

Model Fit Statistics

Log Likelihood	-,625
-2 Log Likelihood	1,251
Akaike's Information Criterion (AIC)	7,251
Hurvich and Tsai's Criterion (AICC)	7,978
Schwarz's Bayesian Criterion (BIC)	12,083

AFT Model Regression Parameters

Parameter	Coefficient	Std. Error	Chi-Squared[a]	Sig.	95% Confidence Interval		Exp. Coefficient	Exp. 95% Confidence Interval	
					Lower	Upper		Lower	Upper
Intercept	5,323	,105	2552,199	<,001	5,116	5,529	204,938	166,702	251,944
group	,130	,066	3,838	,050	,000	,259	1,138	1,000	1,296
(Scale)[b]	,190	,025	.	.	,146	,245	.	.	.

a. Degrees of freedom = 1
b. Chi-squared statistic, p-value, and the exponential statistics are not estimated for the scale parameter.

14.6 Accelerated Failure Time (AFT) Model with Exponential Distribution

The output sheets provide the results from the exponential AFT analysis.

Model Summary

Data Format	Nonrecurrent
Survival Time	time
Model	Accelerated failure time (AFT)
Model Distribution	Exponential
Feature Selection	None
Status	event
ADMM	Fast
Estimation Method	Automatically determined by the procedure

Model Fit Statistics

Log Likelihood	-37,863
-2 Log Likelihood	75,726
Akaike's Information Criterion (AIC)	79,726
Hurvich and Tsai's Criterion (AICC)	80,079
Schwarz's Bayesian Criterion (BIC)	82,947

AFT Model Regression Parameters

Parameter	Coefficient	Std. Error	Chi-Squared[a]	Sig.	95% Confidence Interval		Exp. Coefficient	Exp. 95% Confidence Interval	
					Lower	Upper		Lower	Upper
Intercept	5,400	,556	94,427	<,001	4,311	6,489	221,435	74,510	658,073
group	,090	,348	,067	,795	-,592	,773	1,095	,553	2,166
(Scale)[b]	1,000	.	.	.	.	.	.	.	.

a. Degrees of freedom = 1

b. Scale parameter is fixed at 1 for exponential distribution. Its related statistics are not estimated.

14.7   Accelerated Failure Time (AFT) Model with Log Normal Distribution

The output sheets provide the results from the log normal AFT analysis.

Model Summary

Data Format	Nonrecurrent
Survival Time	time
Model	Accelerated failure time (AFT)
Model Distribution	Log-normal
Feature Selection	None
Status	event
ADMM	Fast
Estimation Method	Automatically determined by the procedure

Model Fit Statistics

Log Likelihood	,309
-2 Log Likelihood	-,617
Akaike's Information Criterion (AIC)	5,383
Hurvich and Tsai's Criterion (AICC)	6,110
Schwarz's Bayesian Criterion (BIC)	10,216

AFT Model Regression Parameters

| Parameter | Coefficient | Std. Error | Chi-Squared[a] | Sig. | 95% Confidence Interval | | Exp. Coefficient | Exp. 95% Confidence Interval | |
					Lower	Upper		Lower	Upper
Intercept	5,291	,116	2098,036	<,001	5,064	5,517	198,459	158,254	248,879
group	,085	,072	1,382	,240	-,057	,227	1,089	,945	1,255
(Scale)[b]	,216	,027	.	.	,170	,276	.	.	.

a. Degrees of freedom = 1

b. Chi-squared statistic, p-value, and the exponential statistics are not estimated for the scale parameter.

14.8   Accelerated Failure Time (AFT) Model with Log Logistics Distribution

The output sheets provide the results from the log logistic AFT analysis.

Model Summary

Data Format	Nonrecurrent
Survival Time	time
Model	Accelerated failure time (AFT)
Model Distribution	Log-logistic
Feature Selection	None
Status	event
ADMM	Fast
Estimation Method	Automatically determined by the procedure

Model Fit Statistics

Log Likelihood	,554
-2 Log Likelihood	-1,108
Akaike's Information Criterion (AIC)	4,892
Hurvich and Tsai's Criterion (AICC)	5,619
Schwarz's Bayesian Criterion (BIC)	9,725

AFT Model Regression Parameters

Parameter	Coefficient	Std. Error	Chi-Squared[a]	Sig.	95% Confidence Interval		Exp. Coefficient	Exp. 95% Confidence Interval	
					Lower	Upper		Lower	Upper
Intercept	5,280	,109	2367,873	<,001	5,067	5,492	196,316	158,709	242,836
group	,096	,069	1,919	,166	-,040	,232	1,101	,961	1,261
(Scale)[b]	,121	,018	.	.	,091	,161	.	.	.

a. Degrees of freedom = 1

b. Chi-squared statistic, p-value, and the exponential statistics are not estimated for the scale parameter.

14.9   Conclusion

	P – value of one group versus the other	Akaike Information Criterion
Cox	0,141	180,409
Weibull	0,050	7251
Exponential	0,795	79,726
Log normal	0,240	5383
Log logistic	0,166	4892

The AFT Weibull provided the best p-value and the only significant one, also the Weibull Akaike Information Criterion was correspondingly small. The Cox regression was statistically insignificant.

References

Five textbooks complementary to the current production and written by the same authors are
(1) Statistics applied to clinical studies 5th edition, 2012,
(2) Machine learning in medicine a complete overview, 2020,
(3) Regression Analysis in Medical Research, 2nd Edition, 2021,
(4) Quantile regression in Clinical Research, 2021,
(5) Kernel Ridge Regression in Clinical research, 2022,
all of them edited by Springer Heidelberg Germany.

Chapter 15
Effect of Group Membership on Survival

Abstract In 81 patients the group membership was a significant predictor of event at p = 0,013. With the Accelerated failure time model with exponential distribution the p-value fell to 0,005.

15.1 Introduction

There are often clinical arguments to support that group membership may influence survival. However documented proof is often missing. In this chapter the effect on survival group membership will be assessed. Survival can be measured in the form of either a hazard, which is the ratio of deaths and non deaths in a random sample, or as a risk which is the proportion of deaths in the same sample. In this chapter hazard and risk of the same data will be computed in an 81 patient parallel group study using respectively Cox regression and Accelerated failure time models.

15.2 Data Example

The effect of group membership on survival was estimated by KB Armitage in 1994 (www.scirp.org).

Supplementary Information The online version contains supplementary material available at https://doi.org/10.1007/978-3-031-31632-6_15.

T. J. Cleophas, A. H. Zwinderman, *Modern Survival Analysis in Clinical Research*, https://doi.org/10.1007/978-3-031-31632-6_15

Group	Time	Event (yes or no, 1 or 0) days
1,00	6,00	1,00
1,00	19,00	1,00
1,00	32,00	1,00
1,00	42,00	1,00
1,00	42,00	1,00
1,00	43,00	,00
1,00	94,00	1,00
1,00	126,00	,00
1,00	169,00	,00
1,00	207,00	1,00
1,00	211,00	,00
1,00	227,00	,00
1,00	253,00	1,00
1,00	255,00	,00
1,00	270,00	,00
1,00	310,00	,00
1,00	316,00	,00
1,00	335,00	,00
1,00	346,00	,00
2,00	4,00	1,00
2,00	6,00	1,00
2,00	10,00	1,00
2,00	11,00	1,00
2,00	11,00	1,00
2,00	11,00	1,00
2,00	13,00	1,00
2,00	17,00	1,00
2,00	20,00	1,00
2,00	20,00	1,00
2,00	21,00	1,00
2,00	22,00	1,00
2,00	24,00	1,00
2,00	24,00	1,00
2,00	29,00	1,00
2,00	30,00	1,00
2,00	30,00	1,00
2,00	31,00	1,00
2,00	33,00	1,00
2,00	34,00	1,00
2,00	35,00	1,00
2,00	39,00	1,00

(continued)

Group	Time	Event (yes or no, 1 or 0) days
2,00	40,00	1,00
2,00	41,00	,00
2,00	43,00	,00
2,00	45,00	1,00
2,00	46,00	1,00
2,00	50,00	1,00
2,00	56,00	1,00
2,00	61,00	,00
2,00	61,00	,00
2,00	63,00	1,00
2,00	68,00	1,00
2,00	82,00	1,00
2,00	85,00	1,00
2,00	88,00	1,00
2,00	89,00	1,00
2,00	90,00	1,00
2,00	93,00	1,00
2,00	104,00	1,00
2,00	110,00	1,00
2,00	134,00	1,00
2,00	137,00	1,00
2,00	160,00	,00
2,00	169,00	1,00
2,00	171,00	1,00
2,00	173,00	1,00
2,00	175,00	1,00
2,00	184,00	1,00
2,00	201,00	1,00
2,00	222,00	1,00
2,00	235,00	,00
2,00	247,00	,00
2,00	260,00	,00
2,00	284,00	,00
2,00	290,00	,00
2,00	291,00	,00
2,00	302,00	,00
2,00	304,00	,00
2,00	341,00	,00
2,00	345,00	,00

15.3   Data Analysis Using SPSS Statistical Software Version 29

The commands for Cox regression and for Accelerated failure time models are summarized underneath.

For convenience the data file entitled "Chapter 15,……" is in SpringerLink supplementary files. Start by opening the data file in your computer mounted with SPSS statistical software version 29.

For Cox regression click in the SPSS Menu:

Analyze….Survival….Cox Regression….time: enter time to event….status: enter event yes or no (1 or 0)….Define Event: enter 1….Covariates….click Categorical….Categorical Covariates: enter covariate….click Continue….click Plots….mark Survival….mark Hazard….click Continue….click OK.
For Accelerated failure times models click:

Analyze….Survival….Parametric Accelerated Failure Times (AFT) Models…. mark Survival….enter: "time" or "follow up mths" or "timetoevent"….status: enter event….click Define Event…default values are given: Failure/Event = 1, Right Censoring = 0, Left Censoring and Interval Censoring are not defined…. click Continue….Covariate(s) enter treatment, age, gender, etc….click Model: mark Distribution of Survival Time….mark Weibull….click Continue…. click OK.

In the output sheets several tables of the goodness of fit and p-values of statistical significance of various covariates are included.

15.4   Cox Regression

With Cox regression hazards and hazard ratios are computed (see also the Chap. 2). Also the Akaike Information Criterion (AIC) is computed. It is an important estimator the goodness of fit of a statistical analysis model. The smaller the AIC value the better the goodness of fit of the data. More information of the AICs (Akaike Information Criteria) as measure for goodness of fit of the analytical model is in the Chap. 2 and many subsequent Chaps. With Cox regression AIC is not computed by SPSS statistical software. But it can be easily calculated using the omnibus tests of coefficients as shown underneath for the data from our data example. Using the commands from the above Sect. 15.3 the computer will provide in the output sheets the underneath tables. The group membership is a significant predictor of survival at p = 0,013.

Omnibus Tests of Model Coefficients

-2 Log Likelihood
415,110

Omnibus Tests of Model Coefficients[a]

-2 Log Likelihood	Overall (score)			Change From Previous Step			Change From Previous Block		
	Chi-square	df	Sig.	Chi-square	df	Sig.	Chi-square	df	Sig.
407,475	6,683	1	,010	7,634	1	,006	7,634	1	,006

a. Beginning Block Number 1. Method = Enter

Variables in the Equation

	B	SE	Wald	df	Sig.	Exp(B)
group	,961	,386	6,210	1	,013	2,614

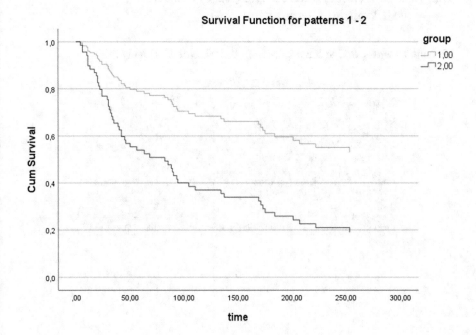

Survival Function for patterns 1 - 2

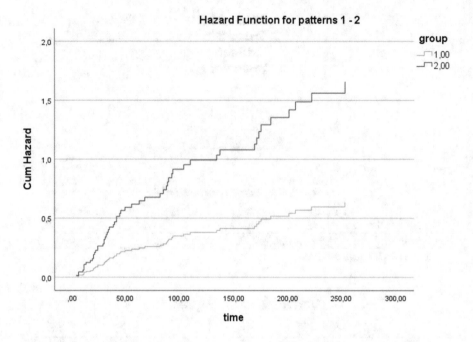

15.5   Accelerated Failure Time (AFT) Models with Weibull Distribution

He output sheets provide the results from the Weibull AFT analysis.

Model Summary

Data Format	Nonrecurrent
Survival Time	time
Model	Accelerated failure time (AFT)
Model Distribution	Weibull
Feature Selection	None
Status	event
ADMM	Fast
Estimation Method	Automatically determined by the procedure

Model Fit Statistics

Log Likelihood	-122,153
-2 Log Likelihood	244,306
Akaike's Information Criterion (AIC)	250,306
Hurvich and Tsai's Criterion (AICC)	250,621
Schwarz's Bayesian Criterion (BIC)	257,452

AFT Model Regression Parameters

Parameter	Coefficient	Std. Error	Chi-Squared[a]	Sig.	95% Confidence Interval		Exp. Coefficient	Exp. 95% Confidence Interval	
					Lower	Upper		Lower	Upper
Intercept	7,386	,892	68,625	<,001	5,639	9,134	1613,659	281,099	9263,253
group	-1,232	,472	6,811	,009	-2,158	-,307	,292	,116	,736
(Scale)[b]	1,208	,136	.	.	,969	1,507	.	.	.

a. Degrees of freedom = 1

b. Chi-squared statistic, p-value, and the exponential statistics are not estimated for the scale parameter.

15.6 Accelerated Failure Time (AFT) Model with Exponential Distribution

The output sheets provide the results from the exponential AFT analysis.

Model Summary

Data Format	Nonrecurrent
Survival Time	time
Model	Accelerated failure time (AFT)
Model Distribution	Exponential
Feature Selection	None
Status	event
ADMM	Fast
Estimation Method	Automatically determined by the procedure

Model Fit Statistics

Log Likelihood	-123,689
-2 Log Likelihood	247,378
Akaike's Information Criterion (AIC)	251,378
Hurvich and Tsai's Criterion (AICC)	251,534
Schwarz's Bayesian Criterion (BIC)	256,142

AFT Model Regression Parameters

Parameter	Coefficient	Std. Error	Chi-Squared[a]	Sig.	95% Confidence Interval		Exp. Coefficient	Exp. 95% Confidence Interval	
					Lower	Upper		Lower	Upper
Intercept	7,109	,722	96,852	<,001	5,693	8,524	1222,319	296,724	5035,191
group	-1,085	,383	8,028	,005	-1,836	-,335	,338	,159	,716
(Scale)[b]	1,000	.	.	.	.	.	.	.	.

a. Degrees of freedom = 1

b. Scale parameter is fixed at 1 for exponential distribution. Its related statistics are not estimated.

15.7   Accelerated Failure Time (AFT) Model with Log Normal Distribution

The output sheets provide the log normal AFT analysis.

Model Summary

Data Format	Nonrecurrent
Survival Time	time
Model	Accelerated failure time (AFT)
Model Distribution	Log-normal
Feature Selection	None
Status	event
ADMM	Fast
Estimation Method	Automatically determined by the procedure

Model Fit Statistics

Log Likelihood	-118,768
-2 Log Likelihood	237,536
Akaike's Information Criterion (AIC)	243,536
Hurvich and Tsai's Criterion (AICC)	243,852
Schwarz's Bayesian Criterion (BIC)	250,682

AFT Model Regression Parameters

Parameter	Coefficient	Std. Error	Chi-Squared[a]	Sig.	95% Confidence Interval		Exp. Coefficient	Exp. 95% Confidence Interval	
					Lower	Upper		Lower	Upper
Intercept	6,544	,811	65,072	<,001	4,954	8,133	694,769	141,697	3406,602
group	-1,087	,438	6,165	,013	-1,945	-,229	,337	,143	,795
(Scale)[b]	1,484	,152	.	.	1,214	1,814	.	.	.

a. Degrees of freedom = 1

b. Chi-squared statistic, p-value, and the exponential statistics are not estimated for the scale parameter.

15.8   Accelerated Failure Time (AFT) Model with Log Logistics Distribution

The output sheets provide the log logistic AFT analysis.

Model Summary

Data Format	Nonrecurrent
Survival Time	time
Model	Accelerated failure time (AFT)
Model Distribution	Log-logistic
Feature Selection	None
Status	event
ADMM	Fast
Estimation Method	Automatically determined by the procedure

Model Fit Statistics

Log Likelihood	-119,521
-2 Log Likelihood	239,042
Akaike's Information Criterion (AIC)	245,042
Hurvich and Tsai's Criterion (AICC)	245,358
Schwarz's Bayesian Criterion (BIC)	252,188

AFT Model Regression Parameters

Parameter	Coefficient	Std. Error	Chi-Squared[a]	Sig.	95% Confidence Interval		Exp. Coefficient	Exp. 95% Confidence Interval	
					Lower	Upper		Lower	Upper
Intercept	6,806	,851	63,900	<,001	5,137	8,475	903,138	170,232	4791,436
group	-1,239	,458	7,327	,007	-2,136	-,342	,290	,118	,710
(Scale)[b]	,878	,099	.	.	,703	1,095			

a. Degrees of freedom = 1

b. Chi-squared statistic, p-value, and the exponential statistics are not estimated for the scale parameter.

15.9   Conclusion

	P-value of significance of difference between one group and the other	Akaike Information Criterion
Cox	0,013,	407,477
Weibull	0,009,	250,306
Exponential	0,005,	251,378
Log normal	0,013,	243,536
Log logistics	0,007	245,358

All of the Accelerated failure time (AFT) models provided better goodness of fit statistics than did the Cox regression. Three of the four AFT models provided better significance of difference between the two groups.

References

Five textbooks complementary to the current production and written by the same authors are
(1) Statistics applied to clinical studies 5th edition, 2012,
(2) Machine learning in medicine a complete overview, 2020,
(3) Regression Analysis in Medical Research, 2nd Edition, 2021,
(4) Quantile regression in Clinical Research, 2021,
(5) Kernel Ridge Regression in Clinical research, 2022,
all of them edited by Springer Heidelberg Germany.

Chapter 16
Multiple Variables Regression Study of 2421 Stroke Patients Assessed for Time to Second Stroke

Abstract In 2421 stroke patients smoking and physical activities were significant predictors of time to second stroke with p-values of 0,001 and 0,05 in the Cox regression. With Accelerated failure time models with log logistics distribution the p-values changed into 0,001 and 0,018 respectively. The data file was available from the "samples" site as attached to SPSS statistical software.

16.1 Introduction and Data Example

There are often clinical arguments to support that multiple covariates may influence a study outomce like survival. However documented proof is often missing. In this chapter the effect on survival of six possible predictors will be first assessed. Survival can be measured in the form of either a hazard, which is the ratio of deaths and non deaths in a random sample, or as a risk which is the proportion of deaths in the same sample. In this chapter hazard and risk of the same data will be computed in a 2421 patient parallel groups study using respectively Cox regression and Accelerated failure time models.

Datafile from "samples" as attached to SPSS statistical software will be used. In a multiple variables Cox regression of 2421 stroke patients with time to second stroke as outcome, two of the six covariates were statistically insignificant predictors, three provided a trend to significance at $0,05 < p < 0,10$, and one provided a p-value of significance at $p = 0,001$.

Supplementary Information The online version contains supplementary material available at https://doi.org/10.1007/978-3-031-31632-6_16.

T. J. Cleophas, A. H. Zwinderman, *Modern Survival Analysis in Clinical Research*, https://doi.org/10.1007/978-3-031-31632-6_16

The p-values are underneath.

Gender	p = 0,3
Physical activities	p = 0,063
Obesity	p = 0,231
Diabetes	p = 0,069
Smoker	p = 0001
Angina	p = 0,054

Of a reduced data model with two instead of six covariates further survival analyses will be performed. The two covariates included as predictors will be smoking and physically active. In all of the analyses both Cox regressions and Accelerated failure time models will be performed.

16.2   Data Analysis in SPSS Statistical Software Version 29

The commands for Cox regression and for Accelerated failure time models are summarized underneath.

For convenience the data file entitled "Chapter 16,……" is in SpringerLink supplementary files. Start by opening the data file in your computer mounted with SPSS statistical software version 29.

For Cox regression click in the SPSS Menu:

Analyze….Survival….Cox Regression….time: enter time to event….status: enter event yes or no (1 or 0)….Define Event: enter 1….Covariates….click Categorical….Categorical Covariates: enter covariate….click Continue….click Plots….mark Survival….mark Hazard….click Continue….click OK.

For Accelerated failure times models click:

Analyze….Survival….Parametric Accelerated Failure Times (AFT) Models…. mark Survival….enter: "time" or "follow up mths" or "timetoevent"….status: enter event….click Define Event…default values are given: Failure/Event = 1, Right Censoring = 0, Left Censoring and Interval Censoring are not defined…. click Continue….Covariate(s) enter treatment, age, gender, etc….click Model: mark Distribution of Survival Time….mark Weibull….click Continue…. click OK.

In the output sheets tables are included of the goodness of fit (Akaike Information Criteria, see also the Chap. 3) and p-values of statistical significance of various covariates.

16.3 Cox Regression

After stepping down and removing insignificant covariates from the data according to:

first step	1 gender, 2 obesity,3 cholesterol
second step	1 afibrillation, 2 history of angina
third step	1 diabetes,

two predictors were left, namely smoking and physically active.

With Cox regression hazards and hazard ratios are computed (see also the Chap. 2). Also the Akaike Information Criterion (AIC) is computed. It is an important estimator the goodness of fit of a statistical analysis model. The smaller the AIC value the better the goodness of fit of the data. More information of the AICs (Akaike Information Criteria) as measure for goodness of fit of the analytical model is in the Chap. 2 and many subsequent Chaps. With Cox regression AIC is not computed by SPSS statistical software. But it can be easily calculated using the omnibus tests of coefficients as shown underneath for the data from our data example. Using the commands from the above Sect. 16.3 the computer provides in the output sheets the underneath tables. Smoking and physically active were indeed independent predictors of survival at p = 0,001 and p = 0,05. Also two Kaplan-Meier curves are in the output sheets.

Categorical Variable Codings[a,c]

		Frequency	(1)
Physically active[b]	0=No	1178	0
	1=Yes	1243	1
Smoker[b]	0=No	1942	0
	1=Yes	479	1

a. Category variable: Physically active (active)

b. Indicator Parameter Coding

c. Category variable: Smoker (smoker)

Omnibus Tests of Model Coefficients

-2 Log Likelihood
35224,024

Omnibus Tests of Model Coefficients[a]

-2 Log Likelihood	Overall (score)			Change From Previous Step			Change From Previous Block		
	Chi-square	df	Sig.	Chi-square	df	Sig.	Chi-square	df	Sig.
35206,020	18,631	2	<,001	18,004	2	<,001	18,004	2	<,001

a. Beginning Block Number 1. Method = Enter

Variables in the Equation

	B	SE	Wald	df	Sig.	Exp(B)
Physically active	-,080	,041	3,852	1	,050	,923
Smoker	,199	,051	15,155	1	<,001	1,220

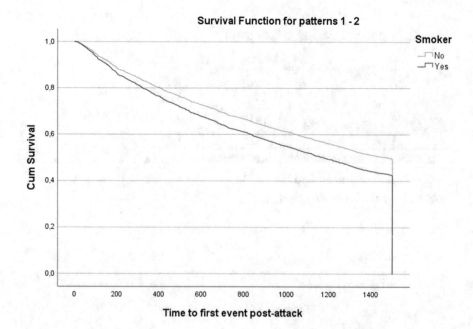

Survival Function for patterns 1 - 2

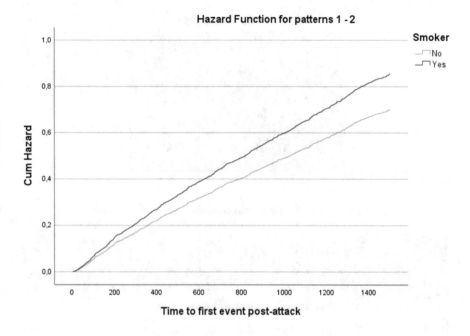

16.4   Accelerated Failure Time (AFT) with Weibull Distribution

The output sheets provide the results from the Weibull AFT analysis.

Model Summary

Data Format	Nonrecurrent
Survival Time	time1
Model	Accelerated failure time (AFT)
Model Distribution	Weibull
Feature Selection	None
Status	VAR00001
ADMM	Fast
Estimation Method	Automatically determined by the procedure

Model Fit Statistics

Log Likelihood	-2714,911
-2 Log Likelihood	5429,822
Akaike's Information Criterion (AIC)	5437,822
Hurvich and Tsai's Criterion (AICC)	5437,838
Schwarz's Bayesian Criterion (BIC)	5460,989

AFT Model Regression Parameters

Parameter	Coefficient	Std. Error	Chi-Squared[a]	Sig.	95% Confidence Interval		Exp. Coefficient	Exp. 95% Confidence Interval	
					Lower	Upper		Lower	Upper
Intercept	7,041	,018	161796,713	<,001	7,006	7,075	1142,264	1103,741	1182,131
smoker	-,095	,029	11,031	<,001	-,151	-,039	,909	,860	,962
active	,044	,023	3,668	,055	-,001	,088	1,045	,999	1,092
(Scale)[b]	,561	,010	.	.	,541	,582	.	.	.

a. Degrees of freedom = 1

b. Chi-squared statistic, p-value, and the exponential statistics are not estimated for the scale parameter.

16.5   Accelerated Failure Time (AFT) with Exponential Distribution

The output sheets provides the results from the exponential AFT analysis.

Model Summary

Data Format	Nonrecurrent
Survival Time	time1
Model	Accelerated failure time (AFT)
Model Distribution	Exponential
Feature Selection	None
Status	VAR00001
ADMM	Fast
Estimation Method	Automatically determined by the procedure

Model Fit Statistics

Log Likelihood	-3127,663
-2 Log Likelihood	6255,325
Akaike's Information Criterion (AIC)	6261,325
Hurvich and Tsai's Criterion (AICC)	6261,335
Schwarz's Bayesian Criterion (BIC)	6278,701

AFT Model Regression Parameters

Parameter	Coefficient	Std. Error	Chi-Squared[a]	Sig.	95% Confidence Interval		Exp. Coefficient	Exp. 95% Confidence Interval	
					Lower	Upper		Lower	Upper
Intercept	6,940	,031	51058,183	<,001	6,880	7,000	1032,651	972,323	1096,721
smoker	-,124	,051	5,899	,015	-,224	-,024	,883	,799	,976
active	,056	,041	1,872	,171	-,024	,135	1,057	,976	1,145
(Scale)[b]	1,000								

a. Degrees of freedom = 1

b. Scale parameter is fixed at 1 for exponential distribution. Its related statistics are not estimated.

16.6   Accelerated Failure Time (AFT) with Log Normal Distribution

The output sheets provide the results from the log normal AFT analysis.

Model Summary

Data Format	Nonrecurrent
Survival Time	time1
Model	Accelerated failure time (AFT)
Model Distribution	Log-normal
Feature Selection	None
Status	VAR00001
ADMM	Fast
Estimation Method	Automatically determined by the procedure

Model Fit Statistics

Log Likelihood	-3361,986
-2 Log Likelihood	6723,972
Akaike's Information Criterion (AIC)	6731,972
Hurvich and Tsai's Criterion (AICC)	6731,989
Schwarz's Bayesian Criterion (BIC)	6755,140

AFT Model Regression Parameters

Parameter	Coefficient	Std. Error	Chi-Squared[a]	Sig.	95% Confidence Interval		Exp. Coefficient	Exp. 95% Confidence Interval	
					Lower	Upper		Lower	Upper
Intercept	6,657	,030	49931,737	<,001	6,599	6,716	778,585	734,422	825,404
smoker	-,192	,050	15,038	<,001	-,289	-,095	,825	,749	,909
active	,063	,039	2,581	,108	-,014	,141	1,065	,986	1,151
(Scale)[b]	,970	,014			,943	,998			

a. Degrees of freedom = 1

b. Chi-squared statistic, p-value, and the exponential statistics are not estimated for the scale parameter.

16.7 Accelerated Failure Time (AFT) with Log Logistic Distribution

The output sheets provide the results from the log logistic AFT analysis.

Model Summary

Data Format	Nonrecurrent
Survival Time	time1
Model	Accelerated failure time (AFT)
Model Distribution	Log-logistic
Feature Selection	None
Status	VAR00001
ADMM	Fast
Estimation Method	Automatically determined by the procedure

Model Fit Statistics

Log Likelihood	-3222,719
-2 Log Likelihood	6445,439
Akaike's Information Criterion (AIC)	6453,439
Hurvich and Tsai's Criterion (AICC)	6453,455
Schwarz's Bayesian Criterion (BIC)	6476,606

AFT Model Regression Parameters

Parameter	Coefficient	Std. Error	Chi-Squared[a]	Sig.	95% Confidence Interval		Exp. Coefficient	Exp. 95% Confidence Interval	
					Lower	Upper		Lower	Upper
Intercept	6,826	,026	68154,174	<,001	6,774	6,877	921,119	875,106	969,551
smoker	-,180	,044	16,564	<,001	-,267	-,093	,835	,766	,911
active	,081	,034	5,553	,018	,014	,148	1,084	1,014	1,159
(Scale)[b]	,496	,009			,479	,513			

a. Degrees of freedom = 1

b. Chi-squared statistic, p-value, and the exponential statistics are not estimated for the scale parameter.

16.8   Conclusion

AIC = Akaike Information Criterion, AFT = Accelerated Failure Time

	AIC	p-values of difference yes/no	
		Smoker	Physically active
Cox	35206,024	0,001	0,05
AFT Weibull	5437,822	0,001	0,055
AFT Exponential	6261,325	0,015	0,171
AFT Log normal	6731,972	0,001	0,108
AFT Log logistics	6453,437	0,001	0,018

The AFT Log logistic model produced the best fit predictive model with p = 0,001 and 0,018 for "smoking" and "physically active". respectively. The p-value of 0,018 was better-sensitive than any other AFT p-value. The Cox model produced pretty good results as well: p-values of p = 0,001 and 0,05 respectively.

References

Five textbooks complementary to the current production and written by the same authors are
(1) Statistics applied to clinical studies 5th edition, 2012,
(2) Machine learning in medicine a complete overview, 2020,
(3) Regression Analysis in Medical Research, 2nd Edition, 2021,
(4) Quantile regression in Clinical Research, 2021,
(5) Kernel Ridge Regression in Clinical research, 2022,
all of them edited by Springer Heidelberg Germany.

Chapter 17
Hypothesized 55 Patient Study of Effect of Treatment Modality on Survival

Abstract In 55 patients treatment modality was an insignificant predictor of event with a p-value of 0,149. With the Accelerated failure time model with log logistics distribution the p-value fell to p = 0,024.

17.1 Introduction

In a hypothesized data-example the effect of treatment modality on event will be assessed. There are often clinical arguments to support that medical treatments may influence survival. However documented proof is often missing. In this chapter the effect on survival of a novel treatment will be assessed against a control treatment. Survival can be measured in the form of either a hazard, which is the ratio of deaths and non deaths in a random sample, or as a risk which is the proportion of deaths in the same sample. In this chapter hazard and risk of the same data will be computed in a 55 patient parallel group study using respectively Cox regression and Accelerated failure time models.

17.2 Data Example

In a hypothesized data example the effect of treatment modality on event was assessed.

Supplementary Information The online version contains supplementary material available at https://doi.org/10.1007/978-3-031-31632-6_17.

155

T. J. Cleophas, A. H. Zwinderman, *Modern Survival Analysis in Clinical Research*, https://doi.org/10.1007/978-3-031-31632-6_17

Time to event (months)	Status event or not	Treatment Modality
2,00	1,00	2,00
2,00	1,00	2,00
4,00	1,00	2,00
4,00	1,00	2,00
6,00	1,00	2,00
8,00	1,00	2,00
2,00	1,00	1,00
3,00	1,00	1,00
5,00	,00	1,00
7,00	1,00	1,00
7,00	1,00	1,00
8,00	1,00	1,00
2,00	1,00	2,00
2,00	1,00	2,00
4,00	1,00	2,00
4,00	1,00	2,00
6,00	1,00	2,00
8,00	1,00	2,00
2,00	1,00	1,00
3,00	1,00	1,00
5,00	,00	1,00
7,00	1,00	1,00
7,00	1,00	1,00
8,00	1,00	1,00
2,00	1,00	2,00
2,00	1,00	2,00
4,00	1,00	2,00
4,00	1,00	2,00
6,00	1,00	2,00
8,00	1,00	2,00
2,00	1,00	1,00
3,00	1,00	1,00
5,00	,00	1,00
7,00	1,00	1,00
7,00	1,00	1,00
8,00	1,00	1,00
2,00	1,00	2,00
2,00	1,00	2,00
4,00	1,00	2,00
4,00	1,00	2,00
6,00	1,00	2,00
8,00	1,00	2,00

(continued)

Time to event (months)	Status event or not	Treatment Modality
2,00	1,00	1,00
3,00	1,00	1,00
5,00	,00	1,00
7,00	1,00	1,00
7,00	1,00	1,00
8,00	1,00	1,00
2,00	1,00	2,00
2,00	1,00	2,00
4,00	1,00	2,00
4,00	1,00	2,00
6,00	1,00	2,00
8,00	1,00	2,00

17.3   Data Analysis Using SPSS Statistical Software Version 29

The commands for Cox regression and for Accelerated failure time models are summarized underneath.

For convenience the data file entitled "Chapter 17,......" is in SpringerLink supplementary files. Start by opening the data file in your computer mounted with SPSS statistical software version 29.

For Cox regression click in the SPSS Menu:

Analyze….Survival….Cox Regression….time: enter time to event….status: enter event yes or no (1 or 0)….Define Event: enter 1….Covariates….click Categorical….Categorical Covariates: enter covariate….click Continue….click Plots….mark Survival….mark Hazard….click Continue….click OK.

For Accelerated failure times models click:

Analyze….Survival….Parametric Accelerated Failure Times (AFT) Models…. mark Survival….enter: "time" or "follow up mths" or "timetoevent"….status: enter event….click Define Event…default values are given: Failure/Event = 1, Right Censoring = 0, Left Censoring and Interval Censoring are not defined…. click Continue….Covariate(s) enter treatment, age, gender, etc….click Model: mark Distribution of Survival Time….mark Weibull….click Continue…. click OK.

In the output sheets AIC (Akaike Information Criterion) tables of the goodness of fit and p-values of statistical significance of various covariates are included.

17.4   Cox Regression

Cox regression is performed using the commands from the Sect. 17.3.

The output sheets underneath provide the results from the Cox regression. With Cox regression hazards and hazard ratios are computed (see also the Chap. 2). Also the Akaike Information Criterion (AIC) is computed. It is an important estimator of the the goodness of fit of a statistical analytic model. The smaller the AIC value the better the goodness of fit of the data. More information of the AICs (Akaike Information Criteria) as measure for goodness of fit of the analytical model is in the Chap. 2 and many subsequent Chaps. With Cox regression AIC is not computed by SPSS statistical software. But it can be easily calculated using the omnibus tests of coefficients (see Chap. 2). The treatment modality was an insignificant predictor of survival at p = 0,149 in the Cox regression.

Kaplan-Meier curves are added.

Omnibus Tests of Model Coefficients

-2 Log Likelihood
328,665

Omnibus Tests of Model Coefficients[a]

-2 Log Likelihood	Overall (score)			Change From Previous Step			Change From Previous Block		
	Chi-square	df	Sig.	Chi-square	df	Sig.	Chi-square	df	Sig.
326,539	2,109	1	,146	2,126	1	,145	2,126	1	,145

a. Beginning Block Number 1. Method = Enter

Variables in the Equation

	B	SE	Wald	df	Sig.	Exp(B)
group	,425	,294	2,081	1	,149	1,529

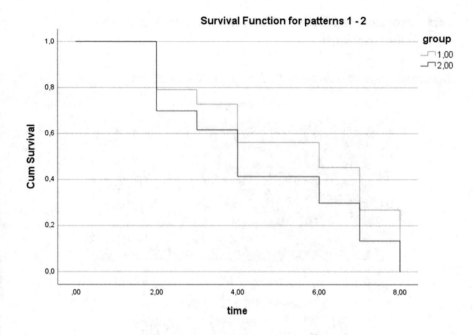

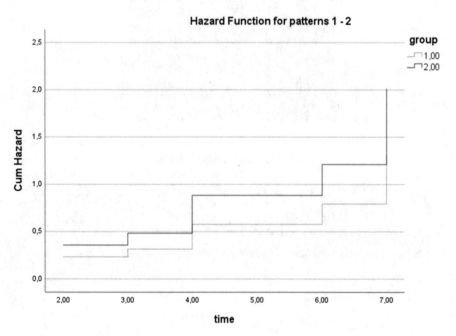

17.5   Accelerated Failure Time (AFT) with Weibull's Distribution

The output sheets provide the rsults from the Weibull AFT analysis.

Model Summary

Data Format	Nonrecurrent
Survival Time	time
Model	Accelerated failure time (AFT)
Model Distribution	Weibull
Feature Selection	None
Status	event
ADMM	Fast
Estimation Method	Automatically determined by the procedure

Model Fit Statistics

Log Likelihood	-40,313
-2 Log Likelihood	80,625
Akaike's Information Criterion (AIC)	86,625
Hurvich and Tsai's Criterion (AICC)	87,105
Schwarz's Bayesian Criterion (BIC)	92,592

AFT Model Regression Parameters

Parameter	Coefficient	Std. Error	Chi-Squared[a]	Sig.	95% Confidence Interval Lower	95% Confidence Interval Upper	Exp. Coefficient	Exp. 95% Confidence Interval Lower	Exp. 95% Confidence Interval Upper
Intercept	2,097	,206	103,166	<,001	1,693	2,502	8,145	5,434	12,208
group	-,245	,124	3,890	,049	-,489	-,002	,782	,613	,998
(Scale)[b]	,427	,049			,341	,534			

a. Degrees of freedom = 1

b. Chi-squared statistic, p-value, and the exponential statistics are not estimated for the scale parameter.

17.6   Accelerated Failure Time (AFT) with Exponential Distribution

The output sheets provide the results from the exponential AFT analysis.

Model Summary

Data Format	Nonrecurrent
Survival Time	time
Model	Accelerated failure time (AFT)
Model Distribution	Exponential
Feature Selection	None
Status	event
ADMM	Fast
Estimation Method	Automatically determined by the procedure

Model Fit Statistics

Log Likelihood	-59,914
-2 Log Likelihood	119,827
Akaike's Information Criterion (AIC)	123,827
Hurvich and Tsai's Criterion (AICC)	124,062
Schwarz's Bayesian Criterion (BIC)	127,805

AFT Model Regression Parameters

Parameter	Coefficient	Std. Error	Chi-Squared[a]	Sig.	95% Confidence Interval		Exp. Coefficient	Exp. 95% Confidence Interval	
					Lower	Upper		Lower	Upper
Intercept	2,246	,483	21,624	<,001	1,300	3,193	9,452	3,667	24,362
group	-,390	,289	1,825	,177	-,956	,176	,677	,385	1,192
(Scale)[b]	1,000	.	.	.	.	.	.	.	.

a. Degrees of freedom = 1

b. Scale parameter is fixed at 1 for exponential distribution. Its related statistics are not estimated.

17.7   Acccelerated Failure Time (AFT) with Log Normal Distribution

The output sheets provide the results from the log normal AFT analysis.

Model Summary

Data Format	Nonrecurrent
Survival Time	time
Model	Accelerated failure time (AFT)
Model Distribution	Log-normal
Feature Selection	None
Status	event
ADMM	Fast
Estimation Method	Automatically determined by the procedure

Model Fit Statistics

Log Likelihood	-42,139
-2 Log Likelihood	84,279
Akaike's Information Criterion (AIC)	90,279
Hurvich and Tsai's Criterion (AICC)	90,759
Schwarz's Bayesian Criterion (BIC)	96,246

AFT Model Regression Parameters

Parameter	Coefficient	Std. Error	Chi-Squared[a]	Sig.	95% Confidence Interval Lower	95% Confidence Interval Upper	Exp. Coefficient	Exp. 95% Confidence Interval Lower	Exp. 95% Confidence Interval Upper
Intercept	1,931	,245	62,024	<,001	1,450	2,411	6,893	4,263	11,144
group	-,296	,149	3,965	,046	-,588	-,005	,744	,556	,995
(Scale)[b]	,533	,053	.	.	,438	,648	.	.	.

a. Degrees of freedom = 1

b. Chi-squared statistic, p-value, and the exponential statistics are not estimated for the scale parameter.

17.8   Accelerated Failure Time (AFT) with Log Logistic Distribution

The output sheets provide the results from the log logistic AFT analysis.

Model Summary

Data Format	Nonrecurrent
Survival Time	time
Model	Accelerated failure time (AFT)
Model Distribution	Log-logistic
Feature Selection	None
Status	event
ADMM	Fast
Estimation Method	Automatically determined by the procedure

Model Fit Statistics

Log Likelihood	-44,320
-2 Log Likelihood	88,641
Akaike's Information Criterion (AIC)	94,641
Hurvich and Tsai's Criterion (AICC)	95,121
Schwarz's Bayesian Criterion (BIC)	100,608

AFT Model Regression Parameters

Parameter	Coefficient	Std. Error	Chi-Squared[a]	Sig.	95% Confidence Interval Lower	95% Confidence Interval Upper	Exp. Coefficient	Exp. 95% Confidence Interval Lower	Exp. 95% Confidence Interval Upper
Intercept	2,067	,263	61,741	<,001	1,552	2,583	7,905	4,720	13,239
group	-,360	,160	5,089	,024	-,674	-,047	,697	,510	,954
(Scale)[b]	,323	,037	.	.	,258	,404	.	.	.

a. Degrees of freedom = 1

b. Chi-squared statistic, p-value, and the exponential statistics are not estimated for the scale parameter.

17.9   Conclusion

	P-value of difference between treatments	Akaike information criterion
Cox	0,149	326,541
AFT Weibull	0,049	86,625
Exponential	0,177	123,827
Log normal	0,046	90,279
Log logistics	0,024	94,641

The best fit AFT (Accelerated failure time) models were found in the Weibull, Log normal, and Log logistic distributions. The Cox regression did not provide a statistically significant result.

References

Five textbooks complementary to the current production and written by the same authors are
(1) Statistics applied to clinical studies 5th edition, 2012,
(2) Machine learning in medicine a complete overview, 2020,
(3) Regression Analysis in Medical Research, 2nd Edition, 2021,
(4) Quantile regression in Clinical Research, 2021,
(5) Kernel Ridge Regression in Clinical research, 2022,
all of them edited by Springer Heidelberg Germany.

Chapter 18
One Year Follow-Up Study with Many Censored Patients

Abstract In a 198 patient one year follow-up study with many censored patients the group membership was an insignificant predictor of deaths at a p-value of p = 0,300. With the Accelerated failure time models p-values repeatedly fell to p = 0,021.

18.1 Introduction

Survival analysis has two types of patients stopping participation. One is death or any other event, the other is stopping participation for any reason but not an event. A censored patient is a patient whose days in the study is accounted but no event is counted in the outcome. In this chapter's data example many censored patients and few events will be observed.

With Cox regression hazards and hazard ratios are computed (see also the Chap. 2). Also the Akaike Information Criterion (AIC) as main estimator of the goodness of fit of a statistical analytic model. The smaller the AIC value, the better the goodness of fit of the data. More information of the AICs (Akaike Information Criteria) as measure for goodness of fit is in the Chap. 2. SPSS statistical software does not provide Cox AICs in the Cox module. Fortunately, they can be easily computed using the omnibus tests of coefficients as shown underneath (see also Chap. 2).

18.2 Data Example

The data of a 198 patient one year follow-up study with many censored patients are underneath. The censored patients are named ,00. The event patients are named 1,00.

Supplementary Information The online version contains supplementary material available at https://doi.org/10.1007/978-3-031-31632-6_18.

time	censored	group
1,00	,00	1,00
,50	,00	1,00
,50	1,00	1,00
1,00	,00	1,00
1,00	,00	1,00
1,00	,00	2,00
1,00	,00	2,00
,50	,00	2,00
1,00	1,00	2,00
1,00	,00	2,00
1,00	,00	2,00
1,00	,00	1,00
,50	,00	1,00
,50	1,00	1,00
1,00	,00	1,00
1,00	,00	1,00
1,00	,00	2,00
1,00	,00	2,00
,50	,00	2,00
1,00	1,00	2,00
1,00	,00	2,00
1,00	,00	2,00
1,00	,00	1,00
,50	,00	1,00
,50	1,00	1,00
1,00	,00	1,00
1,00	,00	1,00
1,00	,00	2,00
1,00	,00	2,00
,50	,00	2,00
1,00	1,00	2,00
1,00	,00	2,00
1,00	,00	2,00
1,00	,00	1,00
,50	,00	1,00
,50	1,00	1,00
1,00	,00	1,00
1,00	,00	1,00
1,00	,00	2,00
1,00	,00	2,00
,50	,00	2,00
1,00	1,00	2,00
1,00	,00	2,00

(continued)

time	censored	group
1,00	,00	2,00
1,00	,00	1,00
,50	,00	1,00
,50	1,00	1,00
1,00	,00	1,00
1,00	,00	1,00
1,00	,00	2,00
1,00	,00	2,00
,50	,00	2,00
1,00	1,00	2,00
1,00	,00	2,00
1,00	,00	2,00
1,00	,00	1,00
,50	,00	1,00
,50	1,00	1,00
1,00	,00	1,00
1,00	,00	1,00
1,00	,00	2,00
1,00	,00	2,00
,50	,00	2,00
1,00	1,00	2,00
1,00	,00	2,00
1,00	,00	2,00
1,00	,00	1,00
,50	,00	1,00
,50	1,00	1,00
1,00	,00	1,00
1,00	,00	1,00
1,00	,00	2,00
1,00	,00	2,00
,50	,00	2,00
1,00	1,00	2,00
1,00	,00	2,00
1,00	,00	2,00
1,00	,00	1,00
,50	,00	1,00
,50	1,00	1,00
1,00	,00	1,00
1,00	,00	1,00
1,00	,00	2,00
1,00	,00	2,00
,50	,00	2,00
1,00	1,00	2,00

(continued)

time	censored	group
1,00	,00	2,00
1,00	,00	2,00
1,00	,00	1,00
,50	,00	1,00
,50	1,00	1,00
1,00	,00	1,00
1,00	,00	1,00
1,00	,00	2,00
1,00	,00	2,00
,50	,00	2,00
1,00	1,00	2,00
1,00	,00	2,00
1,00	,00	2,00
1,00	,00	1,00
,50	,00	1,00
,50	1,00	1,00
1,00	,00	1,00
1,00	,00	1,00
1,00	,00	2,00
1,00	,00	2,00
,50	,00	2,00
1,00	1,00	2,00
1,00	,00	2,00
1,00	,00	2,00
1,00	,00	1,00
,50	,00	1,00
,50	1,00	1,00
1,00	,00	1,00
1,00	,00	1,00
1,00	,00	2,00
1,00	,00	2,00
,50	,00	2,00
1,00	1,00	2,00
1,00	,00	2,00
1,00	,00	2,00
1,00	,00	1,00
,50	,00	1,00
,50	1,00	1,00
1,00	,00	1,00
1,00	,00	1,00
1,00	,00	2,00
1,00	,00	2,00
,50	,00	2,00

(continued)

time	censored	group
1,00	1,00	2,00
1,00	,00	2,00
1,00	,00	2,00
1,00	,00	1,00
,50	,00	1,00
,50	1,00	1,00
1,00	,00	1,00
1,00	,00	1,00
1,00	,00	2,00
1,00	,00	2,00
,50	,00	2,00
1,00	1,00	2,00
1,00	,00	2,00
1,00	,00	2,00
1,00	,00	1,00
,50	,00	1,00
,50	1,00	1,00
1,00	,00	1,00
1,00	,00	1,00
1,00	,00	2,00
1,00	,00	2,00
,50	,00	2,00
1,00	1,00	2,00
1,00	,00	2,00
1,00	,00	2,00
1,00	,00	1,00
,50	,00	1,00
,50	1,00	1,00
1,00	,00	1,00
1,00	,00	1,00
1,00	,00	2,00
1,00	,00	2,00
,50	,00	2,00
1,00	1,00	2,00
1,00	,00	2,00
1,00	,00	2,00
1,00	,00	1,00
,50	,00	1,00
,50	1,00	1,00
1,00	,00	1,00
1,00	,00	1,00
1,00	,00	2,00
1,00	,00	2,00

(continued)

time	censored	group
,50	,00	2,00
1,00	1,00	2,00
1,00	,00	2,00
1,00	,00	2,00
1,00	,00	1,00
,50	,00	1,00
,50	1,00	1,00
1,00	,00	1,00
1,00	,00	1,00
1,00	,00	2,00
1,00	,00	2,00
,50	,00	2,00
1,00	1,00	2,00
1,00	,00	2,00
1,00	,00	2,00
1,00	,00	1,00
,50	,00	1,00
,50	1,00	1,00
1,00	,00	1,00
1,00	,00	1,00
1,00	,00	2,00
1,00	,00	2,00
,50	,00	2,00
1,00	1,00	2,00
1,00	,00	2,00
1,00	,00	2,00

18.3   Data Analysis Using SPSS Statistical Software Version 29

The commands for Cox regression and for Accelerated failure time models are summarized below.

For convenience the data file entitled "Chapter 18,……" is in SpringerLink supplementary files. Start by opening the data file in your computer mounted with SPSS statistical software version 29.

For Cox regression click in the SPSS Menu:

Analyze….Survival….Cox Regression….time: enter time to event….status: enter event yes or no (1 or 0)….Define Event: enter 1….Covariates….click Categorical….Categorical Covariates: enter covariate….click Continue….click Plots….mark Survival….mark Hazard….click Continue….click OK.

For Accelerated failure times models click:

Analyze....Survival....Parametric Accelerated Failure Times (AFT) Models....
mark Survival....enter: "time" or "follow up mths" or "timetoevent"....status:
enter event....click Define Event...default values are given: Failure/Event = 1,
Right Censoring = 0, Left Censoring and Interval Censoring are not defined....
click Continue....Covariate(s) enter treatment, age, gender, etc....click Model:
mark Distribution of Survival Time....mark Weibull....click Continue....
click OK.

In the output sheets several tables of the goodness of fit and p-values of statistical
significance of various covariates are included.

18.4 Cox Regression

Survival will be measured in the form of either a hazard, which is the ratio of deaths
and non deaths in a random sample, or as a risk which is the proportion of deaths in
the same sample. In this chapter hazard and risk will be computed using for the
purpose respectively Cox regression and Accelerated failure time models. The output sheets underneath provide the results from a Cox regression analysis, that can be
obtained from the commands as given in the above Sect. 18.3. The group membership was an insignificant predictor of survival at p = 0,300.

Omnibus Tests of Model Coefficients

-2 Log Likelihood
369,291

Omnibus Tests of Model Coefficients[a]

-2 Log Likelihood	Overall (score)			Change From Previous Step			Change From Previous Block		
	Chi-square	df	Sig.	Chi-square	df	Sig.	Chi-square	df	Sig.
368,222	1,084	1	,298	1,069	1	,301	1,069	1	,301

a. Beginning Block Number 1. Method = Enter

Variables in the Equation

	B	SE	Wald	df	Sig.	Exp(B)
group	-,347	,334	1,074	1	,300	,707

18.5 Accelerated Failure Time (AFT) with Weibull Distribution

The output sheets provide the results of the Weibull's AFT analysis

Model Summary

Data Format	Nonrecurrent
Survival Time	time
Model	Accelerated failure time (AFT)
Model Distribution	Weibull
Feature Selection	None
Status	status
ADMM	Fast
Estimation Method	Automatically determined by the procedure

Model Fit Statistics

Log Likelihood	-53,471
-2 Log Likelihood	106,941
Akaike's Information Criterion (AIC)	112,941
Hurvich and Tsai's Criterion (AICC)	113,294
Schwarz's Bayesian Criterion (BIC)	119,771

AFT Model Regression Parameters

Parameter	Coefficient	Std. Error	Chi-Squared[a]	Sig.	95% Confidence Interval		Exp. Coefficient	Exp. 95% Confidence Interval	
					Lower	Upper		Lower	Upper
Intercept	2,096	,170	152,279	<,001	1,763	2,429	8,137	5,833	11,352
group	-,244	,106	5,340	,021	-,451	-,037	,784	,637	,964
(Scale)[b]	,423	,042	.	.	,348	,514	.	.	.

a. Degrees of freedom = 1

b. Chi-squared statistic, p-value, and the exponential statistics are not estimated for the scale parameter.

18.6   Accelerated Failure Time (AFT) Model with Exponential Distribution

The output sheets provide the results from the exponential AFT analysis.

Model Summary

Data Format	Nonrecurrent
Survival Time	time
Model	Accelerated failure time (AFT)
Model Distribution	Exponential
Feature Selection	None
Status	status
ADMM	Fast
Estimation Method	Automatically determined by the procedure

Model Fit Statistics

Log Likelihood	-79,718
-2 Log Likelihood	159,437
Akaike's Information Criterion (AIC)	163,437
Hurvich and Tsai's Criterion (AICC)	163,611
Schwarz's Bayesian Criterion (BIC)	167,990

AFT Model Regression Parameters

Parameter	Coefficient	Std. Error	Chi-Squared[a]	Sig.	95% Confidence Interval		Exp. Coefficient	Exp. 95% Confidence Interval	
					Lower	Upper		Lower	Upper
Intercept	2,246	,401	31,318	<,001	1,460	3,033	9,452	4,304	20,759
group	-,390	,247	2,488	,115	-,874	,095	,677	,417	1,099
(Scale)[b]	1,000	.	.	.	.	.	.	.	.

a. Degrees of freedom = 1

b. Scale parameter is fixed at 1 for exponential distribution. Its related statistics are not estimated.

18.7   Accelerated Failure Time (AFT) Model with Log Normal Distribution

The output sheets provide the results from the log normal AFT analysis.

Model Summary

Data Format	Nonrecurrent
Survival Time	time
Model	Accelerated failure time (AFT)
Model Distribution	Log-normal
Feature Selection	None
Status	status
ADMM	Fast
Estimation Method	Automatically determined by the procedure

Model Fit Statistics

Log Likelihood	-56,398
-2 Log Likelihood	112,796
Akaike's Information Criterion (AIC)	118,796
Hurvich and Tsai's Criterion (AICC)	119,149
Schwarz's Bayesian Criterion (BIC)	125,626

AFT Model Regression Parameters

Parameter	Coefficient	Std. Error	Chi-Squared[a]	Sig.	95% Confidence Interval		Exp. Coefficient	Exp. 95% Confidence Interval	
					Lower	Upper		Lower	Upper
Intercept	1,931	,205	88,749	<,001	1,529	2,333	6,898	4,615	10,308
group	-,296	,128	5,336	,021	-,548	-,045	,743	,578	,956
(Scale)[b]	,535	,047	.	.	,451	,635	.	.	.

a. Degrees of freedom = 1

b. Chi-squared statistic, p-value, and the exponential statistics are not estimated for the scale parameter.

18.8   Accelerated Failure Time (AFT) Model with Log Logistics Distribution

The output sheets provide the log logistic AFT analysis

Model Summary

Data Format	Nonrecurrent
Survival Time	time
Model	Accelerated failure time (AFT)
Model Distribution	Log-logistic
Feature Selection	None
Status	status
ADMM	Fast
Estimation Method	Automatically determined by the procedure

Model Fit Statistics

Log Likelihood	-112,055
-2 Log Likelihood	224,111
Akaike's Information Criterion (AIC)	230,111
Hurvich and Tsai's Criterion (AICC)	230,235
Schwarz's Bayesian Criterion (BIC)	239,976

AFT Model Regression Parameters

| Parameter | Coefficient | Std. Error | Chi-Squared[a] | Sig. | 95% Confidence Interval | | Exp. Coefficient | Exp. 95% Confidence Interval | |
					Lower	Upper		Lower	Upper
Intercept	-,194	,333	,341	,559	-,847	,458	,823	,429	1,581
group	,384	,207	3,443	,064	-,022	,790	1,469	,979	2,204
(Scale)[b]	,717	,000	.	.	,717	,717	.	.	.

a. Degrees of freedom = 1

b. Chi-squared statistic, p-value, and the exponential statistics are not estimated for the scale parameter.

18.9   Conclusion

	P-value of difference Between two patient groups	Akaike Information Criterion
Cox	0,300,	368,224
AFT Weibull	0,021,	12,941
AFT Exponential	0,115,	163,437
AFT Log normal	0,021,	118,796
AFT Log logistics	0,064,	230,111

The best fit p-values were computed in the AFTs Weibull and Log normal distributions with p = 0,021 twice, the best fit Akaike information criterion was in the AFT Weibull distribution. The Cox regression was very insignificant.

References

Five textbooks complementary to the current production and written by the same authors are
(1) Statistics applied to clinical studies, 5th edition, 2012,
(2) Machine learning in medicine a complete overview, 2020,
(3) Regression Analysis in Medical Research, 2nd Edition, 2021,
(4) Quantile Regression in Clinical Research, 2021,
(5) Kernel Ridge Regression in Clinical Research, 2022,
all of them edited by Springer Heidelberg Germany.

Chapter 19
Alcohol Relapse After Detox Program Treated with or Without a Personal Coach

Abstract In 40 patients on alcohol detox program the treatment with a personal coach was an insignificant predictor of alcohol relapse with a p-value of 0,122 in the Cox regression. With the Accelerated failure time model with log normal distribution the p-value fell to 0,048, and became thus statistically significant at $p < 0,050$.

19.1 Introduction

There are often arguments that psychosocial measures may influence time to alcohol relapse in alcoholics. In this chapter the time to alcohol relapse with or without a personal coach will be assessed. Time to relapse can be measured in the form of either a hazard, which is the ratio of patients with and those without personal coach in a random sample, or as a risk which is the proportion of patients with relapse in the same sample. In this chapter hazard and risk of the same data will be computed in a 40 patient parallel group study using respectively Cox regression and Accelerated failure time models.

19.2 Data Example

Forty alcoholics on a alcohol detox program were treated with or without a personal coach. Time to event was time to alcohol relapse.

Supplementary Information The online version contains supplementary material available at https://doi.org/10.1007/978-3-031-31632-6_19.

time weeks	event	group
1,00	1,00	,00
1,00	1,00	,00
2,00	1,00	,00
3,00	1,00	,00
4,00	1,00	,00
4,00	1,00	,00
27,00	1,00	,00
7,00	1,00	,00
9,00	1,00	,00
11,00	1,00	,00
13,00	1,00	,00
25,00	1,00	,00
17,00	1,00	,00
3,00	1,00	,00
22,00	1,00	,00
4,00	1,00	,00
28,00	1,00	,00
30,00	,00	,00
30,00	,00	,00
30,00	,00	,00
2,00	1,00	1,00
5,00	1,00	1,00
6,00	1,00	1,00
6,00	1,00	1,00
8,00	1,00	1,00
9,00	1,00	1,00
10,00	1,00	1,00
14,00	1,00	1,00
15,00	1,00	1,00
17,00	1,00	1,00
19,00	,00	1,00
24,00	1,00	1,00
26,00	1,00	1,00
28,00	1,00	1,00
30,00	,00	1,00
30,00	,00	1,00
30,00	,00	1,00
30,00	,00	1,00
30,00	,00	1,00
30,00	,00	1,00

19.3   Data Analysis Using SPSS Statistical Software Version 29

The commands for Cox regression and for Accelerated failure time models are summarized underneath.

For convenience the data file entitled "Chapter 19,......" is in SpringerLink supplementary files. Start by opening the data file in your computer mounted with SPSS statistical software version 29.

For Cox regression click in the SPSS Menu:

Analyze....Survival....Cox Regression....time: enter time to event....status: enter event yes or no (1 or 0)....Define Event: enter 1....Covariates....click Categorical....Categorical Covariates: enter covariate....click Continue....click Plots....mark Survival....mark Hazard....click Continue....click OK.

For Accelerated failure times models click:

Analyze....Survival....Parametric Accelerated Failure Times (AFT) Models.... mark Survival....enter: "time" or "follow up mths" or "timetoevent"....status: enter event....click Define Event...default values are given: Failure/Event = 1, Right Censoring = 0, Left Censoring and Interval Censoring are not defined.... click Continue....Covariate(s) enter treatment, age, gender, etc.....click Model: mark Distribution of Survival Time....mark Weibull....click Continue.... click OK.

In the output sheets several tables of the goodness of fit and p-values of statistical significance of various covariates are included.

19.4   Cox Regression

A Cox regression will be first performed of the above data. The commands from the above Sect. 19.3 will be applied for the purpose.

With Cox regression hazards and hazard ratios are computed (see also the Chap. 2). Also the Akaike Information Criterion (AIC) is computed. It is an important estimator of the goodness of fit of a statistical analytic model. The smaller the AIC value the better the goodness of fit of the data. More information of the AICs (Akaike Information Criteria) as measure for goodness of fit of the analytical model is in the Chap. 2 and many subsequent Chaps. With Cox regression AIC is not computed by SPSS statistical software. But it can be easily computed using the omnibus tests of coefficients as shown underneath for the data from our data example. The personal coach was an insignificant predictor of alcohol relapse at p = 0,122, in the Cox regression.

Omnibus Tests of Model Coefficients

-2 Log Likelihood
190,157

Omnibus Tests of Model Coefficients[a]

-2 Log Likelihood	Overall (score)			Change From Previous Step			Change From Previous Block		
	Chi-square	df	Sig.	Chi-square	df	Sig.	Chi-square	df	Sig.
187,733	2,461	1	,117	2,424	1	,119	2,424	1	,119

a. Beginning Block Number 1. Method = Enter

Variables in the Equation

	B	SE	Wald	df	Sig.	Exp(B)
group	-,572	,369	2,396	1	,122	,565

19.5   Accelerated Failure Time (AFT) Models with Weibull Distribution

The output sheets provide the results from the Weibull's AFT analysis.

Model Summary

Data Format	Nonrecurrent
Survival Time	weeks
Model	Accelerated failure time (AFT)
Model Distribution	Weibull
Feature Selection	None
Status	relapse
ADMM	Fast
Estimation Method	Automatically determined by the procedure

Model Fit Statistics

Log Likelihood	-58,183
-2 Log Likelihood	116,366
Akaike's Information Criterion (AIC)	122,366
Hurvich and Tsai's Criterion (AICC)	123,033
Schwarz's Bayesian Criterion (BIC)	127,433

AFT Model Regression Parameters

Parameter	Coefficient	Std. Error	Chi-Squared[a]	Sig.	95% Confidence Interval		Exp. Coefficient	Exp. 95% Confidence Interval	
					Lower	Upper		Lower	Upper
Intercept	2,778	,234	141,338	<,001	2,320	3,236	16,090	10,177	25,437
group	,556	,358	2,408	,121	-,146	1,258	1,744	,864	3,520
(Scale)[b]	,954	,149	.	.	,704	1,295	.	.	.

a. Degrees of freedom = 1
b. Chi-squared statistic, p-value, and the exponential statistics are not estimated for the scale parameter.

19.6   Accelerated Failure Times (AFT) Model with Exponential Distribution

The output sheets provide the results from the exponential AFT analysis.

Model Summary

Data Format	Nonrecurrent
Survival Time	weeks
Model	Accelerated failure time (AFT)
Model Distribution	Exponential
Feature Selection	None
Status	relapse
ADMM	Fast
Estimation Method	Automatically determined by the procedure

Model Fit Statistics

Log Likelihood	-58,227
-2 Log Likelihood	116,454
Akaike's Information Criterion (AIC)	120,454
Hurvich and Tsai's Criterion (AICC)	120,778
Schwarz's Bayesian Criterion (BIC)	123,832

AFT Model Regression Parameters

Parameter	Coefficient	Std. Error	Chi-Squared[a]	Sig.	95% Confidence Interval		Exp. Coefficient	Exp. 95% Confidence Interval	
					Lower	Upper		Lower	Upper
Intercept	2,769	,243	130,337	<,001	2,294	3,244	15,941	9,910	25,643
group	,577	,368	2,452	,117	-,145	1,299	1,781	,865	3,666
(Scale)[b]	1,000	.	.	.	.	.	.	.	.

a. Degrees of freedom = 1

b. Scale parameter is fixed at 1 for exponential distribution. Its related statistics are not estimated.

19.7   Accelerated Failure Time (AFT) Model with Log Normal Distribution

The output sheets provide the results from the log normal AFT analysis.

Model Summary

Data Format	Nonrecurrent
Survival Time	weeks
Model	Accelerated failure time (AFT)
Model Distribution	Log-normal
Feature Selection	None
Status	relapse
ADMM	Fast
Estimation Method	Automatically determined by the procedure

Model Fit Statistics

Log Likelihood	-56,979
-2 Log Likelihood	113,959
Akaike's Information Criterion (AIC)	119,959
Hurvich and Tsai's Criterion (AICC)	120,625
Schwarz's Bayesian Criterion (BIC)	125,025

AFT Model Regression Parameters

Parameter	Coefficient	Std. Error	Chi-Squared[a]	Sig.	95% Confidence Interval		Exp. Coefficient	Exp. 95% Confidence Interval	
					Lower	Upper		Lower	Upper
Intercept	2,201	,273	64,817	<,001	1,665	2,737	9,036	5,287	15,442
group	,782	,395	3,916	,048	,007	1,557	2,186	1,007	4,745
(Scale)[b]	1,202	,163	.	.	,921	1,568	.	.	.

a. Degrees of freedom = 1

b. Chi-squared statistic, p-value, and the exponential statistics are not estimated for the scale parameter.

19.8   Accelerated Failure Times (AFT) Model with Log Logistics Distribution

The output sheets provide the results from the log logistic AFT analysis.

Model Summary

Data Format	Nonrecurrent
Survival Time	weeks
Model	Accelerated failure time (AFT)
Model Distribution	Log-logistic
Feature Selection	None
Status	relapse
ADMM	Fast
Estimation Method	Automatically determined by the procedure

Model Fit Statistics

Log Likelihood	-57,729
-2 Log Likelihood	115,458
Akaike's Information Criterion (AIC)	121,458
Hurvich and Tsai's Criterion (AICC)	122,125
Schwarz's Bayesian Criterion (BIC)	126,525

AFT Model Regression Parameters

Parameter	Coefficient	Std. Error	Chi-Squared[a]	Sig.	95% Confidence Interval		Exp. Coefficient	Exp. 95% Confidence Interval	
					Lower	Upper		Lower	Upper
Intercept	2,221	,293	57,540	<,001	1,647	2,795	9,220	5,193	16,368
group	,746	,408	3,342	,068	-,054	1,546	2,109	,948	4,692
(Scale)[b]	,721	,109			,537	,969			

a. Degrees of freedom = 1
b. Chi-squared statistic, p-value, and the exponential statistics are not estimated for the scale parameter.

19.9   Conclusion

	p-value of difference between treatments	Akaike Information Criterion
Cox	0,122,	187,735
Weibull	0,121,	122,266
Expon	0,117,	120,454
Log normal	0,048,	119,959
Log logistics	0,068.	121,458

The best fit analysis-result has been obtained with the Accelerated Failure Time with a Log normal distribution. The Cox regression analysis was not statistically significant.

References

Five textbooks complementary to the current production and written by the same authors are
(1) Statistics applied to clinical studies 5th edition, 2012,
(2) Machine learning in medicine a complete overview, 2020,
(3) Regression Analysis in Medical Research, 2nd Edition, 2021,
(4) Quantile regression in Clinical Research, 2021,
(5) Kernel Ridge Regression in Clinical research, 2022,
all of them edited by Springer Heidelberg Germany.

Chapter 20
Alcohol Relapse After Detox Program with 3 Predictors

Abstract In 40 patients on alcohol detox program the presence of symptoms, the presence of an alcohol anonymous consultant, and the group membership were significant predictors of alcohol relapse with p-values of 0,001, 0,032, and 0,021 in the Cox regression. With the Accelerated failure time model with log normal distribution the p-values fell to respectively 0,001, 0,001, and 0,007.

20.1 Introduction

There are often arguments that (1) the presence of particular symptoms, (2) the presence of an alcohol anonymous consultant, (3) group membership may influence time to alcohol relapse in alcoholics. In this chapter the time to alcohol relapse with or without the above three factors will be assessed in a multiple variables dataset. Time to relapse can be measured in the form of either a hazard, which is the ratio of patients with and those without personal coach in a random sample, or as a risk which is the proportion of patients with relapse in the same sample. In this chapter hazard and risk of the same data will be computed in a 40 patient parallel group study using respectively Cox regression and Accelerated failure time models.

20.2 Data Example

In forty alcoholics on an alcohol detox program the effect on alcohol relapse of three factors was assessed

(1) the presence of particular symptoms,
(2) the presence of an alcohol anonymous consultant,
(3) group membership.

Supplementary Information The online version contains supplementary material available at https://doi.org/10.1007/978-3-031-31632-6_20.

T. J. Cleophas, A. H. Zwinderman, *Modern Survival Analysis in Clinical Research*, https://doi.org/10.1007/978-3-031-31632-6_20

time = time to event = time to alcohol relapse.
aa-coach = alcohol anonymous coach yes 1 or no 0.

time week	event	group	symptoms	aa-coach
1,00	1,00	,00	4,10	,00
1,00	1,00	,00	3,20	,00
2,00	1,00	,00	3,00	,00
3,00	1,00	,00	3,20	,00
4,00	1,00	,00	4,00	,00
4,00	1,00	,00	2,50	,00
27,00	1,00	,00	1,50	1,00
7,00	1,00	,00	3,80	,00
9,00	1,00	,00	4,50	1,00
11,00	1,00	,00	1,80	,00
13,00	1,00	,00	3,20	1,00
25,00	1,00	,00	2,50	,00
17,00	1,00	,00	3,30	,00
3,00	1,00	,00	3,00	,00
22,00	1,00	,00	2,50	1,00
4,00	1,00	,00	3,00	,00
28,00	1,00	,00	1,20	1,00
30,00	,00	,00	1,80	1,00
30,00	,00	,00	1,00	1,00
30,00	,00	,00	1,80	,00
2,00	1,00	1,00	4,80	,00
5,00	1,00	1,00	2,50	,00
6,00	1,00	1,00	4,50	,00
6,00	1,00	1,00	4,00	,00
8,00	1,00	1,00	2,00	,00
9,00	1,00	1,00	3,00	,00
10,00	1,00	1,00	1,20	,00
14,00	1,00	1,00	2,80	,00
15,00	1,00	1,00	3,00	,00
17,00	1,00	1,00	2,50	1,00
19,00	,00	1,00	1,50	1,00
24,00	1,00	1,00	1,50	,00
26,00	1,00	1,00	2,20	,00
28,00	1,00	1,00	3,30	,00
30,00	,00	1,00	1,00	1,00
30,00	,00	1,00	1,50	,00
30,00	,00	1,00	3,50	,00
30,00	,00	1,00	1,40	1,00
30,00	,00	1,00	2,00	1,00
30,00	,00	1,00	1,50	1,00

20.3   Data Analysis Using SPSS Statistical Software Version 29

The commands for Cox regression and for Accelerated failure time models are summarized underneath.

For convenience the data file entitled "Chapter 20,......" is in SpringerLink supplementary files. Start by opening the data file in your computer mounted with SPSS statistical software version 29.

For Cox regression click in the SPSS Menu:

Analyze....Survival....Cox Regression....time: enter time to event....status: enter event yes or no (1 or 0)....Define Event: enter 1....Covariates....click Categorical....Categorical Covariates: enter covariate....click Continue....click Plots....mark Survival....mark Hazard....click Continue....click OK.

For Accelerated failure times models click:

Analyze....Survival....Parametric Accelerated Failure Times (AFT) Models.... mark Survival....enter: "time" or "follow up mths" or "timetoevent"....status: enter event....click Define Event...default values are given: Failure/Event = 1, Right Censoring = 0, Left Censoring and Interval Censoring are not defined.... click Continue....Covariate(s) enter treatment, age, gender, etc.....click Model: mark Distribution of Survival Time....mark Weibull....click Continue.... click OK.

In the output sheets several tables of the goodness of fit and p-values of statistical significance of various covariates are included.

20.4   Cox Regression

Using the commands from the above Sect. 20.3 a Cox regression analysis will be performed. With Cox regression hazards and hazard ratios are computed (see also the Chap. 2). Also the Akaike Information Criterion (AIC) is computed. It is an important estimator of the goodness of fit of a statistical analytic model. The smaller the AIC value the better the goodness of fit of the data. More information of the AICs (Akaike Information Criteria) as measure for goodness of fit of the analytical model is in the Chap. 2 and many subsequent Chaps. With Cox regression AIC is not computed by SPSS statistical software. But it can be easily computed using the omnibus tests of coefficients as shown underneath for the data from our data example. The three factors

(1) symptoms
(2) aa coach
(3) group memberhip

were significant predictors of alcohol relapse at respectively p = 0,001, 0,032, 0,021 in the Cox regression.

Omnibus Tests of Model Coefficients

-2 Log Likelihood
190,157

Omnibus Tests of Model Coefficients[a]

-2 Log Likelihood	Overall (score)			Change From Previous Step			Change From Previous Block		
	Chi-square	df	Sig.	Chi-square	df	Sig.	Chi-square	df	Sig.
163,296	25,474	3	<,001	26,861	3	<,001	26,861	3	<,001

a. Beginning Block Number 1. Method = Enter

Variables in the Equation

	B	SE	Wald	df	Sig.	Exp(B)
symptoms	,754	,222	11,544	1	<,001	2,125
aa	-1,040	,484	4,614	1	,032	,353
group	-,902	,392	5,306	1	,021	,406

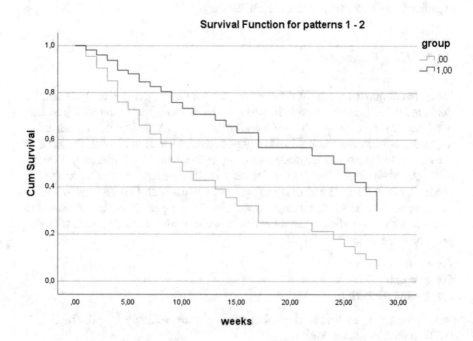

Survival Function for patterns 1 - 2

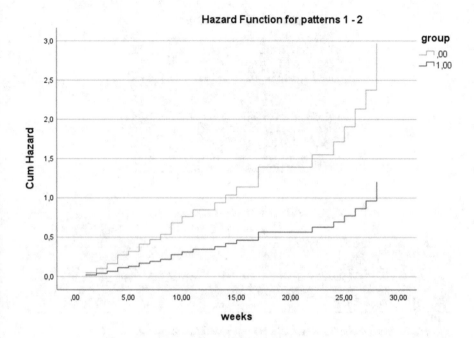

20.5   Accelerated Failure Time (AFT) Model with Weibull Distribution

Model Summary

Data Format	Nonrecurrent
Survival Time	weeks
Model	Accelerated failure time (AFT)
Model Distribution	Weibull
Feature Selection	None
Status	relapse
ADMM	Fast
Estimation Method	Automatically determined by the procedure

Model Fit Statistics

Log Likelihood	-44,216
-2 Log Likelihood	88,433
Akaike's Information Criterion (AIC)	98,433
Hurvich and Tsai's Criterion (AICC)	100,197
Schwarz's Bayesian Criterion (BIC)	106,877

AFT Model Regression Parameters

Parameter	Coefficient	Std. Error	Chi-Squared[a]	Sig.	95% Confidence Interval		Exp. Coefficient	Exp. 95% Confidence Interval	
					Lower	Upper		Lower	Upper
Intercept	3,996	,491	66,323	<,001	3,034	4,958	54,387	20,788	142,288
group	,673	,277	5,883	,015	,129	1,217	1,960	1,138	3,377
symptoms	-,611	,153	15,999	<,001	-,911	-,312	,543	,402	,732
aa	,760	,360	4,468	,035	,055	1,465	2,139	1,057	4,328
(Scale)[b]	,724	,103	.	.	,548	,958	.	.	.

a. Degrees of freedom = 1

b. Chi-squared statistic, p-value, and the exponential statistics are not estimated for the scale parameter.

20.6 Accelerated Failure Time Model with Exponential Distribution

Model Summary

Data Format	Nonrecurrent
Survival Time	weeks
Model	Accelerated failure time (AFT)
Model Distribution	Exponential
Feature Selection	None
Status	relapse
ADMM	Fast
Estimation Method	Automatically determined by the procedure

Model Fit Statistics

Log Likelihood	-46,422
-2 Log Likelihood	92,844
Akaike's Information Criterion (AIC)	100,844
Hurvich and Tsai's Criterion (AICC)	101,987
Schwarz's Bayesian Criterion (BIC)	107,600

AFT Model Regression Parameters

Parameter	Coefficient	Std. Error	Chi-Squared[a]	Sig.	95% Confidence Interval		Exp. Coefficient	Exp. 95% Confidence Interval	
					Lower	Upper		Lower	Upper
Intercept	4,062	,670	36,779	<,001	2,749	5,375	58,100	15,632	215,939
group	,774	,376	4,241	,039	,037	1,511	2,169	1,038	4,533
symptoms	-,675	,202	11,160	<,001	-1,070	-,279	,509	,343	,757
aa	,988	,479	4,247	,039	,048	1,928	2,686	1,050	6,875
(Scale)[b]	1,000								

a. Degrees of freedom = 1

b. Scale parameter is fixed at 1 for exponential distribution. Its related statistics are not estimated.

20.7   Accelerated Failure Time (AFT) with Log Normal Distribution

The output sheets provide the results from the log normal AFT analysis.

Model Summary

Data Format	Nonrecurrent
Survival Time	weeks
Model	Accelerated failure time (AFT)
Model Distribution	Log-normal
Feature Selection	None
Status	relapse
ADMM	Fast
Estimation Method	Automatically determined by the procedure

Model Fit Statistics

Log Likelihood	-40,984
-2 Log Likelihood	81,968
Akaike's Information Criterion (AIC)	91,968
Hurvich and Tsai's Criterion (AICC)	93,732
Schwarz's Bayesian Criterion (BIC)	100,412

AFT Model Regression Parameters

Parameter	Coefficient	Std. Error	Chi-Squared[a]	Sig.	95% Confidence Interval		Exp. Coefficient	Exp. 95% Confidence Interval	
					Lower	Upper		Lower	Upper
Intercept	3,384	,486	48,478	<,001	2,431	4,336	29,483	11,373	76,428
group	,750	,278	7,280	,007	,205	1,295	2,118	1,228	3,653
symptoms	-,574	,144	15,990	<,001	-,855	-,293	,563	,425	,746
aa	1,124	,340	10,951	<,001	,458	1,789	3,076	1,581	5,983
(Scale)[b]	,793	,103			,614	1,024			

a. Degrees of freedom = 1

b. Chi-squared statistic, p-value, and the exponential statistics are not estimated for the scale parameter.

20.8   Accelerated Failure Time (AFT) Model with Log Logistics Distribution

The output sheets provide the results from the log logistic AFT analysis.

Model Summary

Data Format	Nonrecurrent
Survival Time	weeks
Model	Accelerated failure time (AFT)
Model Distribution	Log-logistic
Feature Selection	None
Status	relapse
ADMM	Fast
Estimation Method	Automatically determined by the procedure

Model Fit Statistics

Log Likelihood	-41,457
-2 Log Likelihood	82,914
Akaike's Information Criterion (AIC)	92,914
Hurvich and Tsai's Criterion (AICC)	94,679
Schwarz's Bayesian Criterion (BIC)	101,359

AFT Model Regression Parameters

Parameter	Coefficient	Std. Error	Chi-Squared[a]	Sig.	95% Confidence Interval		Exp. Coefficient	Exp. 95% Confidence Interval	
					Lower	Upper		Lower	Upper
Intercept	3,269	,485	45,516	<,001	2,319	4,218	26,280	10,167	67,926
group	,769	,291	6,983	,008	,199	1,340	2,158	1,220	3,818
symptoms	-,551	,139	15,766	<,001	-,824	-,279	,576	,439	,756
aa	1,144	,332	11,871	<,001	,493	1,795	3,140	1,638	6,021
(Scale)[b]	,459	,069			,342	,617			

a. Degrees of freedom = 1

b. Chi-squared statistic, p-value, and the exponential statistics are not estimated for the scale parameter.

20.9   Conclusion

aa-coach = alcohol anonymous coach
symptoms = sympt = presence of alcohol relapse symptoms or not
Akaike Information = Akaike information criterion

	sympt	aa-coach	group	Akaike Information
Cox	0,01	0,032	0,031,	163,163
Weibull	0,001	0,015	0,035,	98,433
Exponential	0,001	0,039	0,039,	100,844
Log normal	0,001	0,001	0,007	91,968
Log logistics	0,001	0,01	0,008	92,914

The best power of testing has been provided by the log normal and log logistic frequency distributions. Other AFT distributions provided very significant p-values as well.

References

Five textbooks complementary to the current production and written by the same authors are
(1) Statistics applied to clinical studies 5th edition, 2012,
(2) Machine learning in medicine a complete overview, 2020,
(3) Regression Analysis in Medical Research, 2nd Edition, 2021,
(4) Quantile regression in Clinical Research, 2021,
(5) Kernel Ridge Regression in Clinical research, 2022,
all of them edited by Springer Heidelberg Germany.

Chapter 21
Ayurvedic Therapy for Human Immunodeficiency Virus

Abstract In 52 patients with human immunodeficiency virus infection the treatment modality was a significant predictor of the occurrence of neuroaids with a p-value of $p = 0,043$ in the Cox regression. In the Accelerated failure time model with exponential distribution the p-value fell to $p = 0,039$.

21.1 Introduction

In patients with HIV (human immunodeficiency virus) infection neurological complications occurs in 70% of the patients. Ayurvedic therapy mainly consists of herbs and lifestyle treatment, and is common in the ancient Indian system. In this chapter the time to occurrence of neuroaids will be assessed in patients treated with or without ayurvedic therapy. Data will be analyzed with Cox regression and with Accelerated failure time models.

21.2 Data Example

In 52 patients with human immunodeficiency virus infection the treatment modality will be assessed as possibly significant predictor of the occurrence of neuroaids.

Event = occurrence of neuroaids
Treatment = ayurvedic therapy or not

Supplementary Information The online version contains supplementary material available at https://doi.org/10.1007/978-3-031-31632-6_21.

time days	event	treatment (yes or no)
6,00	1,00	1,00
12,00	1,00	1,00
21,00	1,00	1,00
27,00	1,00	1,00
32,00	1,00	1,00
39,00	1,00	1,00
43,00	1,00	1,00
43,00	1,00	1,00
89,00	1,00	1,00
261,00	1,00	1,00
263,00	1,00	1,00
270,00	1,00	1,00
311,00	1,00	1,00
9,00	1,00	2,00
13,00	1,00	2,00
27,00	1,00	2,00
38,00	1,00	2,00
49,00	1,00	2,00
49,00	1,00	2,00
93,00	1,00	2,00
126,00	1,00	2,00
218,00	1,00	2,00
301,00	1,00	2,00
333,00	,00	2,00
369,00	,00	2,00
393,00	,00	2,00
7,00	1,00	1,00
13,00	1,00	1,00
22,00	1,00	1,00
26,00	1,00	1,00
31,00	1,00	1,00
40,00	1,00	1,00
44,00	1,00	1,00
44,00	1,00	1,00
90,00	1,00	1,00
260,00	1,00	1,00
263,00	1,00	1,00
271,00	1,00	1,00
312,00	1,00	1,00
8,00	1,00	2,00
14,00	1,00	2,00

(continued)

time days	event	treatment (yes or no)
28,00	1,00	2,00
37,00	1,00	2,00
50,00	1,00	2,00
49,00	1,00	2,00
92,00	1,00	2,00
125,00	1,00	2,00
219,00	1,00	2,00
302,00	1,00	2,00
332,00	,00	2,00
370,00	,00	2,00
392,00	,00	2,00

21.3   Data Analysis Using SPSS Statistical Software Version 29

The commands for Cox regression and for Accelerated failure time models are summarized underneath.

For convenience the data file entitled "Chapter 21,……" is in SpringerLink supplementary files. Start by opening the data file in your computer mounted with SPSS statistical software version 29.

For Cox regression click in the SPSS Menu:

Analyze….Survival….Cox Regression….time: enter time to event….status: enter event yes or no (1 or 0)….Define Event: enter 1….Covariates….click Categorical….Categorical Covariates: enter covariate….click Continue….click Plots….mark Survival….mark Hazard….click Continue….click OK.

For Accelerated failure times models click:

Analyze….Survival….Parametric Accelerated Failure Times (AFT) Models…. mark Survival….enter: "time" or "follow up mths" or "timetoevent"….status: enter event….click Define Event…default values are given: Failure/Event = 1, Right Censoring = 0, Left Censoring and Interval Censoring are not defined…. click Continue….Covariate(s) enter treatment, age, gender, etc.….click Model: mark Distribution of Survival Time….mark Weibull….click Continue…. click OK.

In the output sheets several tables of the goodness of fit and p-values of statistical significance of various covariates are included.

21.4   Cox Regression

With the help of the commands from the above Sect. 21.3 first a Cox regression will be performed. With Cox regression hazards and hazard ratios are computed (see also the Chap. 2). Also the Akaike Information Criterion (AIC) is computed. It is an important estimator of the goodness of fit of a statistical analytic model. The smaller the AIC value the better the goodness of fit of the data. More information of the AICs (Akaike Information Criteria) as measure for goodness of fit of the analytical model is in the Chap. 2 and many subsequent Chaps. With Cox regression AIC is not computed by SPSS statistical software. But it can be easily computed using the omnibus tests of coefficients as shown underneath for the data from our data example. The treatment modality was a significant predictor of survival at p = 0,043, in the Cox regression.

Omnibus Tests of Model Coefficients

-2 Log Likelihood
300,156

Omnibus Tests of Model Coefficients[a]

-2 Log Likelihood	Overall (score)			Change From Previous Step			Change From Previous Block		
	Chi-square	df	Sig.	Chi-square	df	Sig.	Chi-square	df	Sig.
295,992	4,230	1	,040	4,164	1	,041	4,164	1	,041

a. Beginning Block Number 1. Method = Enter

Variables in the Equation

	B	SE	Wald	df	Sig.	Exp(B)
group	-,614	,303	4,110	1	,043	,541

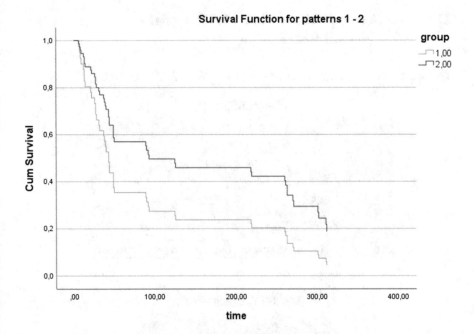

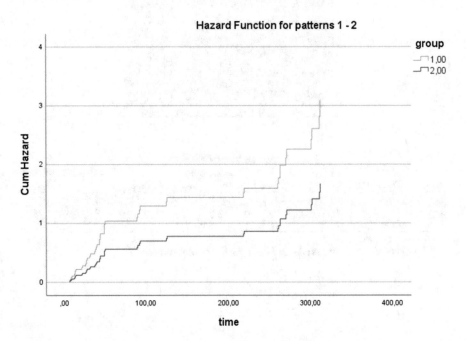

21.5   Accelerated Failure Time (AFT) Model with Weibull Distribution

The output sheets provide the results from the Weibull AFT analysis.

Model Summary

Data Format	Nonrecurrent
Survival Time	time
Model	Accelerated failure time (AFT)
Model Distribution	Weibull
Feature Selection	None
Status	event
ADMM	Fast
Estimation Method	Automatically determined by the procedure

Model Fit Statistics

Log Likelihood	-88,316
-2 Log Likelihood	176,632
Akaike's Information Criterion (AIC)	182,632
Hurvich and Tsai's Criterion (AICC)	183,132
Schwarz's Bayesian Criterion (BIC)	188,486

AFT Model Regression Parameters

Parameter	Coefficient	Std. Error	Chi-Squared[a]	Sig.	95% Confidence Interval		Exp. Coefficient	Exp. 95% Confidence Interval	
					Lower	Upper		Lower	Upper
Intercept	3,923	,550	50,824	<,001	2,845	5,002	50,570	17,197	148,706
group	,680	,359	3,588	,058	-,024	1,384	1,974	,977	3,991
(Scale)[b]	1,197	,142	.	.	,949	1,511	.	.	.

a. Degrees of freedom = 1

b. Chi-squared statistic, p-value, and the exponential statistics are not estimated for the scale parameter.

21.6   Accelerated Failure Time (AFT) Model with Exponential Distribution

The output sheets provide the results from the exponential AFT analysis.

Model Summary

Data Format	Nonrecurrent
Survival Time	time
Model	Accelerated failure time (AFT)
Model Distribution	Exponential
Feature Selection	None
Status	event
ADMM	Fast
Estimation Method	Automatically determined by the procedure

Model Fit Statistics

Log Likelihood	-89,560
-2 Log Likelihood	179,119
Akaike's Information Criterion (AIC)	183,119
Hurvich and Tsai's Criterion (AICC)	183,364
Schwarz's Bayesian Criterion (BIC)	187,022

AFT Model Regression Parameters

Parameter	Coefficient	Std. Error	Chi-Squared[a]	Sig.	95% Confidence Interval		Exp. Coefficient	Exp. 95% Confidence Interval	
					Lower	Upper		Lower	Upper
Intercept	4,080	,451	81,647	<,001	3,195	4,965	59,124	24,404	143,245
group	,614	,297	4,259	,039	,031	1,197	1,847	1,031	3,309
(Scale)[b]	1,000	.	.	.	.	.	.	.	.

a. Degrees of freedom = 1

b. Scale parameter is fixed at 1 for exponential distribution. Its related statistics are not estimated.

21.7   Accelerated Failure Time (AFT) Model with Log Normal Distribution

The output sheets provide the results from the log normal AFT analysis.

Model Summary

Data Format	Nonrecurrent
Survival Time	time
Model	Accelerated failure time (AFT)
Model Distribution	Log-normal
Feature Selection	None
Status	event
ADMM	Fast
Estimation Method	Automatically determined by the procedure

Model Fit Statistics

Log Likelihood	-85,934
-2 Log Likelihood	171,867
Akaike's Information Criterion (AIC)	177,867
Hurvich and Tsai's Criterion (AICC)	178,367
Schwarz's Bayesian Criterion (BIC)	183,721

AFT Model Regression Parameters

Parameter	Coefficient	Std. Error	Chi-Squared[a]	Sig.	95% Confidence Interval		Exp. Coefficient	Exp. 95% Confidence Interval	
					Lower	Upper		Lower	Upper
Intercept	3,458	,602	32,995	<,001	2,278	4,638	31,745	9,756	103,293
group	,572	,384	2,215	,137	-,181	1,324	1,771	,834	3,759
(Scale)[b]	1,365	,146	.	.	1,106	1,684	.	.	.

a. Degrees of freedom = 1

b. Chi-squared statistic, p-value, and the exponential statistics are not estimated for the scale parameter.

21.8   Accelerated Failure Time (AFT) Model with Log Logistics Distribution

The output sheets provide the results from the log logistic AFT analysis.

Model Summary

Data Format	Nonrecurrent
Survival Time	time
Model	Accelerated failure time (AFT)
Model Distribution	Log-logistic
Feature Selection	None
Status	event
ADMM	Fast
Estimation Method	Automatically determined by the procedure

Model Fit Statistics

Log Likelihood	-87,447
-2 Log Likelihood	174,893
Akaike's Information Criterion (AIC)	180,893
Hurvich and Tsai's Criterion (AICC)	181,393
Schwarz's Bayesian Criterion (BIC)	186,747

AFT Model Regression Parameters

Parameter	Coefficient	Std. Error	Chi-Squared[a]	Sig.	95% Confidence Interval Lower	95% Confidence Interval Upper	Exp. Coefficient	Exp. 95% Confidence Interval Lower	Exp. 95% Confidence Interval Upper
Intercept	3,432	,632	29,516	<,001	2,194	4,670	30,938	8,970	106,710
group	,572	,407	1,970	,160	-,227	1,370	1,771	,797	3,934
(Scale)[b]	,827	,099	.	.	,654	1,047	.	.	.

a. Degrees of freedom = 1

b. Chi-squared statistic, p-value, and the exponential statistics are not estimated for the scale parameter.

21.9   Conclusion

	P-value of difference between treatments	Akaike Information Criterion (AIC)
Cox regression	0,043	295,994
Weibull distribution	0,058	182,632
Exponential distribution	0,039	183,110
Log normal distribution	0,137	177,867
Log logistics distribution	0,160	180,893

   The AIC values of the Accelerated failure time models provided much better goodnes of fit than did the AIC of the Cox regression. The p-value of difference between treatment modalities of the AFT Exponential distribution was statistically significant at 0,039, The other three AFT models were not significant. The Cox regression was significant at a p-value of 0,043.

References

Five textbooks complementary to the current production and written by the same authors are
(1) Statistics applied to clinical studies 5th edition, 2012,
(2) Machine learning in medicine a complete overview, 2020,
(3) Regression Analysis in Medical Research, 2nd Edition, 2021,
(4) Quantile regression in Clinical Research, 2021,
(5) Kernel Ridge Regression in Clinical research, 2022,
all of them edited by Springer Heidelberg Germany.

Chapter 22
Time to Event Regressions Other Than Cox Regressions

Abstract Time to event regressions are used to describe the percentages of patients having an event in longitudinal studies. However, in survival studies the numbers of events are often disproportionate with time, or checks are not timely made, or changes are sinusoidally due to seasonal effect. Many more mechanisms may bias exponential-event-like patterns. Examples are given as well as appropriate alternative methods for analyses.

22.1 Introduction

In the current edition traditional proportional hazard regression method of Cox and Accellerated Failure Time models are explained. It is underlined that both methods are based on exponential models with per time unit the same percentage of patients having an event, a pretty strong assumption for complex creatures like human beings. Yet it has been widely used for the assessment of time to event analyses, even if the data do not very well match an exponential model. Some alternative models will be reviewed in this chapter with the help of data examples.

1. Cox with Time Dependent Predictors. Special form of Cox regression first published in reviews by the scientific editor Prentice-Hall NJ 1978.
2. Segmented Cox. Special form of Cox regression first published in reviews by the scientific editor Prentice-Hall NJ 1978.
3. Interval Censored Regressions, one of many generalized linear models with a so-called interval censored link function (see also the Chaps. 4 and 5).

Supplementary Information The online version contains supplementary material available at https://doi.org/10.1007/978-3-031-31632-6_22.

205

T. J. Cleophas, A. H. Zwinderman, *Modern Survival Analysis in Clinical Research*, https://doi.org/10.1007/978-3-031-31632-6_22

4. Linear correlation coefficients for seasonal observations developed by Yule (1871–1951 Tuebingen Germany), Box (1932–1982 London UK), and Jenkins (1919–2013 Madison Wisconsin).
5. Polynomial regression models are usually fit using the method of least squares, as published in 1805 by Legendre (Chap. 1) and in 1809 by Gauss (Chap. 2). The first design of an experiment for polynomial regression appeared in an 1815 paper of Gergonne (1771–1859 Montpellier France).

22.2   Cox with Time Dependent Predictors

Cox regression assumes, that the proportional hazard of a predictor regarding survival works time-independently. However, in practice time-dependent disproportional hazards are not uncommon. E.g., the level of LDL cholesterol is a strong predictor of cardiovascular survival. However, in a survival study virtually no one will die from elevated values in the first decade of observation. LDL cholesterol may be, particularly, a killer in the second decade of observation, and in the third decade those with high levels may all have died, and other reasons for dying may occur. In other words the deleterious effect of 10 years elevated LDL-cholesterol may be different from that of 20 years. The traditional Cox regression model is not appropriate for analyzing the effect of LDL cholesterol on survival, because it assumes that the relative hazard of dying is the same in the first, second and third decade. Thus, there seems to be a time-dependent disproportional hazard, and if you want to analyze such data, an extended Cox regression model allowing for non-proportional hazards must be applied, and is available in SPSS. We will use the underneath data example. The first 10 patients are given in the table underneath. The entire data file is entitled "Chapter 22,1, ……..", and is in SpringerLink supplementary files (treat = treatment modality).

Variables 1-6

time to event	event 1 = yes	treat 0 or 1	age years	gender 0 = fem	LDL-cholesterol 1 = > 3,9 mmol/l
1	2	3	4	5	6
1,00	1	0	65,00	,00	1,00
1,00	1	0	66,00	,00	1,00
2,00	1	0	73,00	,00	1,00
2,00	1	0	54,00	,00	1,00
2,00	1	0	46,00	,00	1,00
2,00	1	0	37,00	,00	1,00
2,00	1	0	54,00	,00	1,00
2,00	1	0	66,00	,00	1,00
2,00	1	0	44,00	,00	1,00
3,00	0	0	62,00	,00	1,00

Start by opening the data file in your computer with SPSS installed. First, a time-independent Cox analysis will be performed.

Command:

Analyze....Survival....Cox Regression....time: follow years....status: event....Define Event: enter 1....Covariates....click Categorical....Categorical Covariates: enter elevated LDL-cholesterol....click Continue....click Plots....mark Survival....mark Hazard....click Continue....click OK.

Variables in the Equation

	B	SE	Wald	df	Sig.	Exp(B)
cholesterol	-,544	,332	2,682	1	,102	,581

Var 00006 is a binary variable for LDL-cholesterol. It is not a significant predictor of survival with a p-value and a hazard ratio of only 0,102 and 0.581 respectively, as demonstrated above by a simple Cox regression with event as outcome variable and LDL cholesterol as predictor. The investigators believe that the presence of LDL-cholesterol must be a determinant of survival. And if we look at the data, we will observe that something very special is going on: in the first decade virtually no one with elevated LDL-cholesterol dies. In the second decade virtually everyone with an elevated LDL-cholesterol does: LDL-cholesterol seems to be particularly a killer in the second decade. Then, in the third decade other reasons for dying seem to have taken over. In order to assess whether elevated LDL-cholesterol adjusted for time has a significant effect on survival, a time-dependent Cox regression will be performed. For that purpose the time–dependent covariate is defined as a function of both the variable time (called "T_" in SPSS) and the LDL-cholesterol variable, while using the product of the two. This product is applied as "time-dependent predictor of survival", and a usual Cox model is, subsequently, performed (Cov = covariate). For analysis the statistical model Cox Time Dependent in the module Survival is required.

Command:

Analyze....Survival....Cox w/Time-Dep Cov....Compute Time-Dep Cov....Time (T_)
  transfer to box Expression for T_Cov....add the sign *....add the LDL-cholesterol
  variable....Model....Time: follow months....Status: event - ?: Define Event: enter
  1....click Continue....T_Cov transfer to box Covariates....click OK.

Variables in the Equation

	B	SE	Wald	df	Sig.	Exp(B)
T_COV_	-,131	,033	15,904	1	,000	,877

The above results table of the "Cox regression with time-dependent variables" shows that the presence of an elevated LDL-cholesterol adjusted for differences in time is a highly significant predictor of survival. Time dependent Cox regression is convenient, if some of your predictors are time dependent, like in the above data example.

22.3   Segmented Cox

Segmented time-dependent Cox regression goes one step further than the above time dependent Cox, and it assesses, whether the interaction with time is different at different periods of the study. An example is given. The primary scientific question: is frailty a time-dependently changing variable in patients admitted to hospital for exacerbation of chronic obstructive pulmonary disease (COPD). A simulated data file of 60 patients admitted to hospital for exacerbation of COPD is given underneath. All of the patients are assessed for frailty scores once a week. The frailty scores run from 0 to 100 (no frail to very frail).

Variables

1	2	3	4	5	6
days discharge	cured	gender	frailty 1st	frailty 2nd	frailty 3rd week

1,00	1,00	1,00	15,00		
1,00	1,00	1,00	18,00		
1,00	1,00	1,00	16,00		
1,00	1,00	1,00	17,00		
2,00	1,00	1,00	15,00		
2,00	1,00	1,00	20,00		
2,00	1,00	1,00	16,00		
2,00	1,00	1,00	15,00		
3,00	1,00	,00	18,00		
3,00	1,00	,00	15,00		
3,00	1,00	1,00	16,00		
4,00	1,00	1,00	15,00		
4,00	1,00	1,00	18,00		
5,00	1,00	1,00	19,00		
5,00	1,00	1,00	19,00		
5,00	1,00	1,00	19,00		
6,00	1,00	1,00	18,00		
6,00	1,00	1,00	17,00		
6,00	1,00	,00	19,00		
7,00	1,00	,00	16,00		
8,00	1,00	,00	60,00	15,00	
8,00	1,00	,00	69,00	16,00	
8,00	1,00	,00	67,00	17,00	
9,00	1,00	1,00	60,00	19,00	
9,00	1,00	1,00	86,00	24,00	
10,00	1,00	1,00	87,00	16,00	
10,00	1,00	,00	75,00	10,00	
10,00	1,00	,00	76,00	20,00	
10,00	1,00	,00	67,00	32,00	
11,00	1,00	1,00	56,00	24,00	
11,00	1,00	1,00	78,00	25,00	
12,00	1,00	1,00	58,00	26,00	
12,00	1,00	,00	59,00	25,00	
13,00	1,00	,00	77,00	20,00	
13,00	1,00	1,00	66,00	16,00	
13,00	1,00	1,00	65,00	18,00	
13,00	1,00	1,00	68,00	10,00	
14,00	1,00	1,00	85,00	16,00	
14,00	1,00	,00	65,00	23,00	
14,00	1,00	,00	65,00	20,00	
15,00	1,00	,00	54,00	60,00	14,00
16,00	1,00	,00	43,00	68,00	15,00

variable 1 = days to discharge from hospital
variable 2 = cured or lost from observation (1 = cured)
variable 3 = gender
variable 4 = frailty index first week (0-100)
variable 5 = frailty index second week (0-100)
variable 6 = frailty index third week (0-100).
The missing values in the variables 5 and 6 are those from patients already discharged from hospital.

The above table gives the first 42 patients of 60 patients assessed for their frailty scores after 1, 2 and 3 weeks of clinical treatment. It can be observed that in the first week frailty scores at discharge were 15–20, in the second week 15–32, and in the third week 14–24. Patients with scores over 32 were never discharged. Frailty scores were probably a major covariate of time to discharge. The entire data file is in SpringerLink supplementary files, and is entitled "Chapter 22, 2, ...". We will first perform a simple time-dependent Cox regression. Start by opening the data file in your computer. For analysis the statistical model Cox Time Dependent in the module Survival is required.

Command:

Analyze....Survival....Cox w/Time-Dep Cov....Compute Time-Dep Cov....Time (T_); transfer to box Expression for T_Cov....add the sign *....add the frailty variable third week....Model....Time: day of discharge....Status: cured or lost.... Define: cured = 1....Continue....T_Cov: transfer to Covariates....click OK.

Variables in the Equation

	B	SE	Wald	df	Sig.	Exp(B)
T_COV_	,000	,001	,243	1	,622	1,000

The above table shows the result: frailty is not a significant predictor of day of discharge. However, patients are generally not discharged from hospital, until they are non-frail at a reasonable level, and this level may be obtained at different periods of time. Therefore, a segmented time dependent Cox regression may be more adequate for analyzing these data.

For analysis the statistical model Cox Time Dependent in the module Survival is again required.

Command:

Survival.....Cox w/Time-Dep Cov....Compute Time-Dependent Covariate....
Expression for T_COV_: enter $(T\_ \geq 1 \,\&\, T\_ < 11) * VAR00004 + (T\_ \geq 11 \,\&\, T\_ < 21) * VAR00005 + (T\_ \geq 21 \,\&\, T\_ < 31)$....Model....Time: enter Var 1.... Status: enter Var 2 (Define events enter 1)....Covariates: enter T_COV_ .... click OK).

Variables in the Equation

	B	SE	Wald	df	Sig.	Exp(B)
T_COV_	-,056	,009	38,317	1	,000	,945

The above table shows that the independent variable, segmented frailty variable T_COV_, is, indeed, a very significant predictor of the day of discharge. We will, subsequently, perform a multiple segmented time dependent Cox regression with treatment modality as second predictor variable. For analysis a multiple segmented time dependent Cox regression must be performed.

Command:

same commands as above, except for Covariates: enter T_COV and treatment....
click OK.

Variables in the Equation

	B	SE	Wald	df	Sig.	Exp(B)
T_COV_	-,060	,009	41,216	1	,000	,942
VAR00003	,354	,096	13,668	1	,000	1,424

The above table shows that both the frailty (variable T_COV_) and treatment
(variable 3) are very significant predictors of the day of discharge with hazard ratios
of 0,942 and 1,424. The new treatment is about 1,4 times better and the patients are
doing about 0,9 times worse per frailty score point.

22.4   Interval Censored Regressions

In survival studies often time to first outpatient clinic check instead of time to event
is measured. Somewhere in the interval between the last and current visit an event
may have taken place. For simplicity such data are often analyzed using the proportional hazard model of Cox. However, this analysis is not entirely appropriate here.
It assumes that time to first outpatient check is equal to time to relapse. Instead of a
time to relapse, an interval is given, in which the relapse has occurred, and so this
variable is somewhat more loose than the usual variable time to event. An appropriate statistic for the current variable would be the mean time to relapse inferenced
from a generalized linear model with an interval censored link function, rather than
the proportional hazard method of Cox.

A data example is given. In 51 patients in remission their status at the time-to-
first-outpatient-clinic-control was checked (mths = months, treat = treatment).

time to 1st check result (month)	treat relapse 0 = no (0 or 1)	modality 1 or 2
11	0	1
12	1	0
9	1	0
12	0	1
12	0	0
12	0	1
5	1	1
12	0	1
12	0	1
12	0	0

The first 10 patients are above. The entire data file is entitled "Chap. 22,3,.....", and is in SpringerLink supplementary files. It is previously used by the authors in SPSS for starters and 2nd levelers, Chap. 59, Springer Heidelberg Germany, 2016. Start by opening the data file in SPSS statistical software. For analysis the module Generalized Linear Models is required. It consists of two submodules: Generalized Linear Models and Generalized Estimation Models. For the censored data analysis the Generalized Linear Models submodule of the Generalized Linear Models module is required.

Command:

Analyze....click Generalized Linear Models....click once again Generalized Linear Models....Type of Model....mark Interval censored survival....click Response.... Dependent Variable: enter Result....Scale Weight Variable: enter "time to first check"....click Predictors....Factors: enter "treatment"....click Model....click once again Model: enter once again "treatment"....click Save....mark Predicted value of mean of response....click OK.

Parameter Estimates

Parameter	B	Std. Error	95% Wald Confidence Interval		Hypothesis Test		
			Lower	Upper	Wald Chi-Square	df	Sig.
(Intercept)	.467	.0735	.323	.611	40.431	1	.000
[treatment=0]	-.728	.1230	-.969	-.487	35.006	1	.000
[treatment=1]	0ᵃ	.	.	.	.	.	.
(Scale)	1ᵇ						

Dependent Variable: Result
Model: (Intercept), treatment

a. Set to zero because this parameter is redundant.
b. Fixed at the displayed value.

The generalized linear model shows, that, after censoring the intervals, the treatment 0 is, as compared to treat 1, a very significant maintainer of remission.

22.5 Autocorrelations

Seasonal data are data that are repetitive by season. The assessment of seasonality requires a measure of repetitiveness. Levels of linear autocorrelation is such a measure. It may not be regression analysis, but linear correlation coefficients are closely related to linear regression. Linear correlation coefficients of the values between slightly different seasonal curves are used for making predictions from seasonal data about the presence of seasonality.

Average C-reactive protein in group of healthy subjects (mg/l)	Month
1,98	1
1,97	2
1,83	3
1,75	4
1,59	5
1,54	6
1,48	7
1,54	8
1,59	9
1,87	10

The entire data file is in SpringerLink supplementary files, and is entitled "Chapter 22, 4,......". It was previously used by the authors in SPSS for starters and 2nd levelers, Chap. 58, Springer Heidelberg Germany, 2016. Start by opening the data file in your computer with SPSS installed.

Command:

Graphs....Chart Builder....click Scatter/Dot....click mean C-reactive protein level and drag to the Y-Axis....click time and drag to the X-Axis....click OK..... double-click in Chart Editor....click Interpolation Line....Properties: click Straight Line.

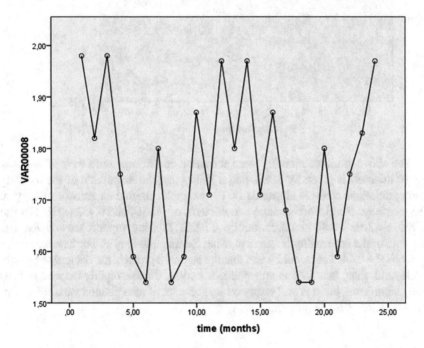

The above graph shows that the average monthly C-reactive protein levels look seasonal.

We will now assess seasonality with autocorrelations.

For analysis the statistical model Autocorrelations in the module Forecasting is required.

Command:

Analyze....Forecasting....Autocorrelations....move monthly percentages into
    Variable Box....mark Autocorrelations....mark Partial Autocorrelations....OK.

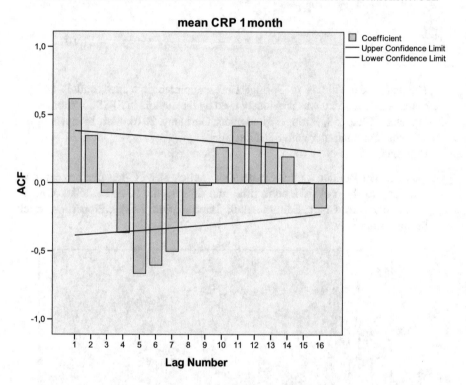

The above graph of monthly autocorrelation coefficients with their 95% confidence intervals is given by SPSS, and it shows that the magnitude of the monthly autocorrelations changes sinusoidally. For example, significant autocorrelations at the month no. 5 and 12 (correlation coefficients of -0.664 and 0.452 (SE $0,174$ and 0.139, t-values -3.80 and 3.25, both $p < 0.001$)) further support seasonality. The strength of the seasonality is assessed using the magnitude of r^2. For example $= r^2 = (-0.664)^2 = 0.44$. This would mean that the lagcurve predicts the datacurve by only 44 %, and, thus, that 56% is unexplained. And so, the seasonality may be statistically significant, but it is still pretty weak, and a lot of unexplained variability, otherwise called noise, is present.

22.6   Polynomial Regressions

Underneath polynomial regression equations of the first to fifth order are given with y as dependent and x as independent variables.

$y = a + bx$	first order (linear) relationship
$y = a + bx + cx^2$	second order (parabolic) relationship
$y = a + bx + cx^2 + dx^3$	third order (hyperbolic) relationship
$y = a + bx + cx^2 + dx^3 + ex^4$	fourth order (sinusoidal) relationship
$y = a + bx + cx^2 + dx^3 + ex^4 + fx^5$	fifth order relationship

Higher order polynomes can visualize longitudinal observations in clinical research.

As an example, in a patient with mild hypertension ambulatory blood pressure measurement was performed using a portable equipment every 30 min for 24 hours. The first 10 measurements are underneath, the entire data file is entitled "Chapter 22, 5", and is in SpringerLink supplementary files. It is previously used by the authors in SPSS for starters and 2nd levelers, Chap. 60, Springer Heidelberg Germany, 2016. Start by opening tha data file in your computer with SPSS installed.

Blood pressure mm Hg	Time (30 min intervals)
205,00	1,00
185,00	2,00
191,00	3,00
158,00	4,00
198,00	5,00
135,00	6,00
221,00	7,00
170,00	8,00
197,00	9,00
172,00	10,00
188,00	11,00
173,00	12,00

SPSS statistical software will be used for polynomial modeling of these data. Open the data file in SPSS. For analysis the module General Linear Model is required. We will use the submodule Univariate here.

Command:

Analyze....General Linear Model....Univariate....Dependent: enter y (mm Hg)....
   Covariate(s): enter x (min)....click: Options....mark: Parameter Estimates....click

Continue....click Paste....in "/Design=x" replace x with a 5th order polynomial equation tail (* is sign of multiplication)

$$x\ x^*x\ x^*x^*x\ x^*x^*x^*x\ x^*x^*x^*x^*x$$

....then click the green triangle in the upper graph row of your screen.

The underneath table is in the output sheets, and gives you the partial regression coefficients (B values) of the 5th order polynomial with blood pressure as outcome and with time as independent variable (–7,135E-6 indicates 0.000007135, which is a pretty small B value. However, in the equation it will have to be multiplied with x^5, and a large, very large term will result even so.

Parameter Estimates

Dependent Variable:y

Parameter	B	Std. Error	t	Sig.	95% Confidence Interval	
					Lower Bound	Upper Bound
Intercept	206,653	17,511	11,801	,000	171,426	241,881
x	-9,112	6,336	-1,438	,157	-21,858	3,634
x*x	,966	,710	1,359	,181	-,463	2,395
x*x*x	-,047	,033	-1,437	,157	-,114	,019
x*x*x*x	,001	,001	1,471	,148	,000	,002
x*x*x*x*x	-7,135E-6	4,948E-6	-1,442	,156	-1,709E-5	2,819E-6

Parameter Estimates

Dependent Variable:yy

Parameter	B	Std. Error	t	Sig.	95% Confidence Interval	
					Lower Bound	Upper Bound
Intercept	170,284	11,120	15,314	,000	147,915	192,654
x	-7,034	4,023	-1,748	,087	-15,127	1,060
x*x	,624	,451	1,384	,173	-,283	1,532
x*x*x	-,027	,021	-1,293	,202	-,069	,015
x*x*x*x	,001	,000	1,274	,209	,000	,001
x*x*x*x*x	-3,951E-6	3,142E-6	-1,257	,215	-1,027E-5	2,370E-6

The entire equations can be written from the above B values:

$$y = 206.653 - 9{,}112x + 0.966x^2 - 0.47x^3 + 0.001x^4 + 0.000007135x^5$$

This equation is entered in the polynomial grapher of David Wees available on the internet at "davidwees.com/polygrapher/", and the underneath graph is drawn. This graph is speculative as none of the x terms is statistically significant. Yet, the actual data have a definite patterns with higher values at daytime and lower ones at night.

sometimes even better fit curve are obtained by taking higher order polynomes like 5th order polynomes. We should add, that, in spite of the insignificant p-values in the above tables, the two polynomes are not meaningless. The first one suggests some white coat effect, the second one suggests normotension and a normal dipping pattern. With machine learning meaningful visualizations can sometimes be produced of your data, even if statistics are pretty meaningless.

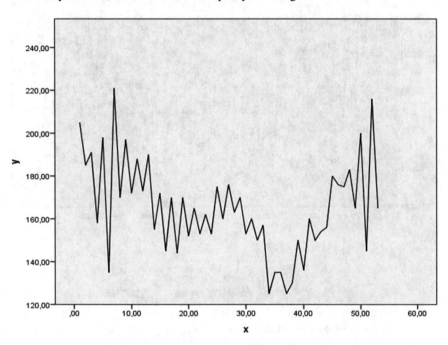

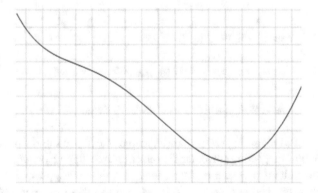

24 hour ABPM recording (30 min measures) of untreated subject with hypertension and 5th order polynome (suggesting some white coat effect).

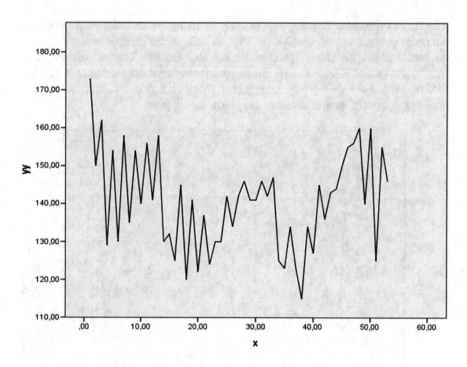

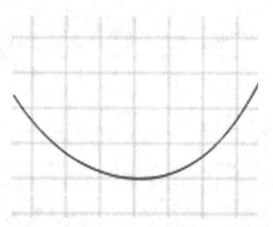

24 hour ABPM recording (30 min measures) of the above subject treated and 5th order polynome (suggesting normotension and a normal dipping pattern). Polynomes of ambulatory blood pressure measurements can thus be applied for visualizing hypertension types and treatment effects, as well as other circadian response patterns in clinical research.

22.7 Conclusion

Cox and Accelerated failure time regressions are based on an exponential model with per time unit the percentage of patients have an event, a pretty strong assumption for complex creatures like human beings. Yet they has been widely used for the assessment of time to event analyses, even if the data do not very well match an exponential model. Alternative models are available. In this chapter the underneath models have been explained with the help of data examples.

1. Cox with Time Dependent Predictors is particularly suitable. Cox regression assumes that the proportional hazard of a predictor regarding survival works time-independently. However, in practice time-dependent disproportional hazards are not uncommon. E.g., the level of LDL cholesterol is a strong predictor of cardiovascular survival. However, in a survival study virtually no one will die from elevated values in the first decade of observation. LDL cholesterol may be, particularly, a killer in the second and third decades of observation.
2. Segmented time-dependent Cox regression goes one step further than the above time dependent Cox, and it assesses, whether the interaction with time is different at different periods of the study.
3. With interval censored regressions, instead of a time to relapse, an interval is given, in which the relapse has occurred, and so this variable is somewhat more loose than the usual variable time to event. An appropriate statistic for the current variable would be the mean time to relapse inferenced from a generalized linear model with an interval censored link function, rather than the proportional hazard method of Cox. However, we should add that also Accelerated failure time (AFT) analysis with interval censoring is possible, and is covered in the SPSS menu for AFTs. A problem is though, that information about start time and end time of observation is required for each patient, which are often missing in Kaplan Meier data.
4. Seasonal data are data that are repetitive by season. The assessment of seasonality requires a measure of repetitiveness. Levels of linear autocorrelation is such a measure. Linear correlation coefficients of the values between slightly different seasonal curves are used for making predictions from seasonal data about the presence of seasonality.
5. Polynomial regression equations of increasing orders with y as dependent time variable and x as predictor variable give linear (= first order) relationship, parabolic (= second order) relationship, hyperbolic (= third order) relationship, sinusoidal (= fourth order) relationship, etc. Higher order polynomes can be used to visualize the effects of predictors like treatments, and patient characteristics, on circadian cardiovascular, hormonal, and other biological rhythms.

References

Five textbooks complementary to the current production and written by the same authors are
(1) Statistics applied to clinical studies 5th edition, 2012,
(2) Machine learning in medicine a complete overview, 2020,
(3) Regression Analysis in Medical Research, 2nd Edition, 2021,
(4) Quantile regression in Clinical Research, 2021,
(5) Kernel Ridge Regression in Clinical research, 2022,
all of them edited by Springer Heidelberg Germany.

Chapter 23
Abstracts of the Chapters 1 to 22

Chapter 1
Students in medicine and health sciences find regression analyses harder than any other methodology in statistics. This edition will start with a brief review of history, and methodologies of regression analyses. Linear regression has a continuous outcome variable. In contrast, logistic and Cox regressions have binary outcomes, and use logarithmic transformations of odds or hazards. This edition will particularly focus on the novel models for survival analysis entitled Accelerated failure times models, that provide generally better data-fit than does the traditional Cox regressions based on odds of events, here otherwise called hazard of events, particularly if the events are nasty.

Chapter 2
The Chaps. 1, 2, and 3 of this edition review the general principles of the most popular regression models in a nonmathematical fashion, including linear regression, the main purposes of regression analyses, the methods of logistic regression for event analysis, and Cox regression for hazard analysis. Cox regression is just like logistic regression immensely popular in clinical research. It is based on an exponential pattern: per time unit the same % of patients has an event.

Chapter 3
Accelerated failure time models do not use, like Cox regression (Chap. 1), the hazard of death, but, rather, the risk of death. The hazard is the ratio "death / non-deaths", while the risk of death is the ratio "death / entire population at the start of a study". The hazard runs from zero to ∞, whereas the risk runs from zero to 1 (=100%). Both hazard and risk modeling can be accomplished with mathematical functions that are even largely similar. For the purpose of optimized fitting the relationships between time and survival-chance, and their relative chances five options may be chosen:

T. J. Cleophas, A. H. Zwinderman, *Modern Survival Analysis in Clinical Research*, https://doi.org/10.1007/978-3-031-31632-6_23

1. Weibull models,
2. Exponential models,
3. Log-normal models,
4. Log-logistic models,
5. Hypertabastic models based on hyperbolic secants (the inverse of hyperbolic cosinuses).

Mathematical models are for finding and fitting significant relationships between predictor and outcome variables. Traditional tests are usually applied for testing how far distant the data are from the best fit models. The closer to one another they are, the better-suited the models are for predictive purposes, like times to event, survival, deaths, failures.

Chapter 4
In 60 patients with cardiovascular disase the treatment modality was a significant predictor of event with a p-value of 0,004 in the Cox regression. With the Accelerated failure fime model the p-value even fell to p = 0,001.

Chapter 5
In this multiple variables predictive model the effect of three predictors on mortality were assessed. The treatment modality and cholesterol were independend predictors both with p-values of 0,001 in the Cox regression. With the Accelerated failure time model with Weibull distribution equal p-values were obtained.

Chapter 6
In 29 patients with glioma brain cancer treatment modality was an insignificant predictor of event with a p-value of 0,083. With the Accelerated failure time model with exponential distribution the p-value fell to 0,047, and became thus statistically significant at p < 0,05.

Chapter 7
In 28 patients with metastatic colonic cancer the treatment modality was a significant predictor of event with a p-value of 0,010 in the Cox regression. With the Accelerated failure time models the best predictive p-value was p = 0,001 which was ten times better than that of the Cox model. For all of the AFT (Accelerated failure time) models the AIC (Akaike Information Criterion) goodness of fit measure was over twice better with AIC values around 25,000 as compared to that of the Cox regression of close to 70,000 (the smaller the value, the better the fit). AFT p-values were correspondingly generally much smaller than those of the Cox regression.

Chapter 8
In 23 patients with acute myeloid leucemia maintained chemotherapy was an insignificant predictor of survival with a p-value of 0,078. With the Accelerated failure time model with a Weibull distribution the p-value feel to 0,015.

Chapter 9
In a 15 patient mortality study the treatment modality was an insignificant predictor of mortality with a p-value of 0,138. With the Accelerated failure time model with Weibull distribution the p-value fell to 0,008.

Chapter 10
In 81 patients with histiocytic lymphoma the disease stage was a significant predictor of survival at a p-value of 0,013 in the Cox regression. With the Accelerated failure time model with exponential distribution the p-value fell to 0,005. The effect of stage on survival was estimated in patients with stage 1 and stage 2 histiocytic lymphoma.

Chapter 11
In 64 lymphoma patients the presence of B symptoms was a significant predictor of survival with a p-value of 0,007 in the Cox regression. In the Accelerated failure time models with both the exponential and the log logistics distributions the p-values fell to 0,001.

Chapter 12
In 18 patients the group membership was an insignificant predictor of event with a p-value of 0,058 in the Cox regression. With the Accelerated failure time model with Weibull distribution the p-value fell to 0,008.

Chapter 13
In 12 patients the group membership was an insignificant predictor of event with a p-value of 0,109 in the Cox regression. With the Accelerated failure time model with a log normal distribution the p-value fell to 0,047, and became thus statistically significant at $p < 0.05$.

Chapter 14
In 38 rats the exposure to carcinogens was an insignificant predictor of deaths from carcinoma with a p-value of 0,141 in the Cox regression. With the Accelerated failure time model with Weibull distribution the p-value fell to 0,050.

Chapter 15
In 81 patients the group membership was a significant predictor of event at $p = 0,013$. With the Accelerated failure time model with exponential distribution the p-value fell to 0,005.

Chapter 16
In 2421 stroke patients smoking and physical activities were significant predictors of time to second stroke with p-values of 0,001 and 0,05 in the Cox regression. With Accelerated failure time models with log logistics distribution the p-values changed into 0,001 and 0,018 respectively. The data file was available from the "samples" site as attached to SPSS statistical software.

Chapter 17

In 55 patients treatment modality was an insignificant predictor of event with a p-value of 0,149. With the Accelerated failure time model with log logistics distribution the p-value fell to p = 0,024.

Chapter 18

In a 198 patient follow up study the group membership was an insignificant predictor of deaths at a p-value of p = 0,300. With the Accelerated failure time model with log normal distribution the p-value fell to p = 0,021.

Chapter 19

In 40 patients on alcohol detox program the treatment with a personal coach was an insignificant predictor of alcohol relapse with a p-value of 0,122 in the Cox regression. With the Accelerated failure time model with log normal distribution the p-value fell to 0,048, and became thus statistically significant at p < 0,050.

Chapter 20

In 40 patients on alcohol detox program the presence of symptoms, the presence of a alcohol anonymous consultant, and the group membership were significant predictors of alcohol relapse with p-values of 0,001, 0,032, and 0,021 in the Cox regression. With the Accelerated failure time model with log normal distribution the p-values fell to respectively 0,001, 0,001, and 0,007.

Chapter 21

In 52 patients with human immunodeficiency virus infection the treatment modality was a significant predictor of the occurance of neuroaids with a p-value of p = 0,043 in the Cox regression. In the Accelerated failure time model with exponential distribution the p-value fell to p = 0,039.

Chapter 22

Time to event regressions are used to describe the percentages of patients having an event in longitudinal studies. However, in survival studies the numbers of events are often disproportionate with time, or checks are not timely made, or changes are sinusoidally due to seasonal effect. Many more mechanisms may bias exponential-event-like patterns. Examples are given as well as appropriate alternative methods for analyses.

References

Five textbooks complementary to the current production and written by the same authors are
(1) Statistics applied to clinical studies 5th edition, 2012,
(2) Machine learning in medicine a complete overview, 2020,
(3) Regression Analysis in Medical Research, 2nd Edition, 2021.
(4) Quantile regression in Clinical Research, 2021.
(5) Kernel Ridge Regression in Clinical research, 2022,
all of them edited by Springer Heidelberg Germany.

Printed in the United States
by Baker & Taylor Publisher Services